LOW BLOOD SUGAR

The Hidden Menace of Hypoglycemia

CLEMENT G. MARTIN, M.D.

A FIRESIDE BOOK
Published by Simon & Schuster
New York London Toronto Sydney Tokyo Singapore

FIRESIDE
Simon & Schuster Building
Rockefeller Center
1230 Avenue of the Americas
New York, New York 10020

Published in 1986 by Prentice Hall Press
First Fireside Edition 1992

Previously published by Arco Publishing, Inc.
by arrangement with Information Incorporated
Original Title: *How To Eat Your Way Out of Fatigue*

Manufactured in the United States of America

23   22   21   20

Library of Congress Catalog Card Number: 74-112735

ISBN 0-671-76410-1

contents

1

Eat Your Way Out of Fatigue

"I GUESS I'm not as young as I once was. I feel tired all the time." A common statement, but one based on a false idea. Healthy aging has no signs, although certain illnesses do tend to show up as we get older. These signs show that there is something wrong with the body machinery. If you know what these signs are you can do something about them—you may need the help of your physician, but in simple cases you may be able to take care of matters yourself.

From age 30 onward, fatigue is frequently a problem, and it is often self-caused. Eating habits formed in youth and early adult life are usually not right for the mature years. We all eat what we like more than we eat what we should. When we start to run out of energy we reach, automatically, for quick-energy foods: sugars and starches. These are—for the moment. They give us the "lifts" that we need, and we feel that we have helped ourselves out of the crisis of fatigue. So begins the vicious circle of fatigue, overweight, and mental confusion that is the too-common lot of many adults in America today. The way out of this problem —the finding of more vitality, better physical health, more mental alertness, is the subject of this book.

Psychosomatic is a long word, and one with more meaning to it than we often realize. The feeling of fatigue, for example, is just as often a mental feeling as it is a physical feeling. Since our brain runs on the same fuel that the rest of our body does, this is not really strange. When our body starts to run out of fuel, it becomes difficult to think, just as it becomes difficult to be physically active. When we have this difficulty in thinking clearly it becomes all the harder to figure out what the source of our trouble is. Are our emotions awry, or is there something wrong with our body? We try to explain our problems to someone else and we can't express them adequately, and knowing this, we feel all the more uncertain and mentally confused. This is the description of a psychosomatic problem. The Psyche—mind, emotion, thought processes—is dependent upon a healthy body—soma. The illness of one is reflected in upset of the other. These disorders usually come on slowly. You are not healthy one day and sick the next in a drastic fashion. The beginnings, and the progress, are insidious. When you begin to feel that these are normal bodily changes that all people experience as they grow older, a feeling of hopelessness is added to your upset. Again, let me emphasize that this is a far from hopeless condition: it is one that is readily corrected. Straightening yourself out is neither going to be difficult nor take any great deal of time. As with much of life, discovering what the problem is is better than half the solution.

The stories of others who have had conditions you may also have experienced often help you to see what your own problems and solutions can be. The story of Tom L. is not at all unusual. He was an energetic and charming man who worked hard and had the admiration of his fellow workers and the executives where he worked. About eight months before I saw him he had had a promotion. He now had more income, more responsibility, and an even better future ahead. But very soon after this step upward in his career he began to feel short of energy. He awoke feeling fine, had his early morning coffee and went to the office filled with energy. But by the ten o'clock coffee break he was nervous and jittery, and added to this he frequently could not get his desired coffee and snack because meetings would progress right through the break. Not getting his necessary "pick-up," he would become irritable and crabby, and attempt to make decisions before he was fully aware of the problems. He really had to have something at this time or his hands would begin to shake; occasionally he'd begin to perspire. This looked, to all concerned, like the failures that frequently occur when a man is promoted over his head and beyond his capacities.

Somehow or another he would drag on until lunchtime. If possible, he would have a quick cocktail before lunch. One was enough—it relaxed him and he suddenly felt that the world wasn't so bad anymore. Then he'd have a "good lunch"—lots of starches, lots of fat, and a very full feeling afterwards. Then Tom was his "old self," happy, joking and brilliant. He'd be eager to get back to work, realizing that really not too much had been done during the morning, and feeling a real desire to straighten out the messes that he had left behind. With all the stuffing inside of him he was a bit logy, but he was mentally alert and could go about his business well. Excellent. Until about 2:30 or 3:00 in the afternoon—coffee break time. Once again, he began to be a little shaky and nervous and to feel awfully tired. Not only were there a few less meetings in the afternoon, but his associates also felt the need for a lift at this time, and coffee was served more regularly. But it didn't help as much as he hoped it would and he still felt tired. To Tom it meant only one thing: he had been over-promoted. This was pretty discouraging news. He wished he could think clearly enough to do something about it.

Fortunately, he realized he couldn't solve the problem all by himself, and he sought medical advice. The routine tests showed "nothing wrong." Routine, whether in medicine or elsewhere, is often not the answer. A little digging was needed to find out where things were wrong. Quick inspection showed that Tom was a little heavier and flabbier than he had been a year before. That's not unusual; but it was different. He did not have the physical strength that he should have had on his fitness test either—but that's even more frequent a finding. Dr. Warren Guild of Harvard Medical School states, quite correctly, that 97 percent of all adult Americans are unfit. But, this was not that simple a problem. There had been changes; there was something wrong. What was it? Something in the body's machinery was out of gear. A test of his carbohydrate metabolism was in order, and a glucose tolerance test (GTT). Not one of those nice, neat one- or two-hour tests, but a nearly all-day affair would be needed to find out what the matter was if, indeed, such a disturbance was the cause. The idea of spending five hours in a laboratory did not appeal to Tom. He knew he was not doing his full job in business and feared that a day away might be bad for his career. But he listened to advice and found a day when he could properly have the test done.

The object of the glucose tolerance test is to demonstrate the body's ability to handle carbohydrate-sugar. This is done in a standardized way so that meaning can be obtained from the tests without much difficulty. The glucose test is always accurate for the time in which the test is being done. Preparation is necessary to insure that the test be valid for you and your body, and special attention must be paid to diet for several days before the test begins. Because of this disease and its symptoms, you may well have been eating in an unusual fashion and must go back to a general diet to be properly prepared for this examination. If a person eats very little, particularly very little carbohydrate, he may have a *starvation* blood sugar test, which looks much like diabetes. People who eat "normally," meaning with sufficient carbohydrates, do not have to do any special preparatory dieting before they take the test, and this was the case with Tom. He was told to eat as he had been up until midnight the night before the test, and then he was to begin fasting. He knew that a number of blood samples were to be taken and that he would get sugary drink, loaded with carbohydrates, to take early in the course of the experiment.

It was well worth his while, for a diagnosis was made. During the first three hours he sat around, read magazines and felt pretty good. During the fourth hour he felt a little tired and everyone agreed this could well be just plain boredom, or annoyance with the test procedure itself.

As the fifth hour approached, Tom began to change visibly. Color drained from his face, his forehead was damp with perspiration, and he began to tremble. The time for the next blood test hadn't arrived yet, but a test was taken as soon as these symptoms became evident. Had he gotten much worse, the test would have been stopped by giving him a drink of orange juice. But he rallied and got rid of the severe shakes. He said his mental condition was still very confused, and he wondered what could be done about this. The fifth hour test was taken, and he was given the orange juice and started to feel better very quickly. Everyone in the lab felt a lot better; a diagnosis had been established for Tom's problem. He had hypoglycemia—low blood sugar. This condition, the opposite of diabetes, was the source of all his problems, both mental and physical—psychosomatic.

The reason for Tom's symptoms was a sudden insufficiency of sugar, blood glucose, in his bloodstream. This put all of his body's mechanisms under a severe stress. His perspiring and chill was a symptom of this stress. His mental confusion was a direct result of the brain's inability to run without sugar. Had he had any difficulty with the circulation around his heart, this stress could have produced a heart attack! Hypoglycemia is often the final insult that wrecks a heart already burdened with hardened arteries. Some physicians have pointed out that heart attacks are most frequent four or five hours after eating heavy meals, and attribute these episodes to hypoglycemia.

Shirley M., now 37 years old, had been an attractive, gay student and later a community leader. She had advanced degrees from universities, and three attractive children. But her life seemed empty. Her once stunning figure had disappeared under considerable layers of fat. Reading the daily paper was now an effort—she just couldn't focus her mind on it long enough. She could rarely recall what yesterday's news had been. She thought she might have a solution to the whole mess—suicide.

On taking a detailed history, it was evident that her troubles had started about five years ago. Since her youngest child was eight years old, it was obvious that pregnancies were not the cause of her difficulties. She didn't seem like a hypoglycemia patient; several other diagnoses seemed much more plausible. The routine tests were made, and a few of the fancier ones as well; nothing showed up. Well, was she just a "mess" the way she said she was? It didn't seem likely; underneath all this confusion and weight there was a person in trouble. She was also given the five-hour glucose toler-ance test.

She went through the test with no trouble at all. No sweating, no chills, no increased weakness, but she had a positive test. Her blood sugar went to a value of about 50, well below the normal range. She did not have enough energy to operate as a normal person. The rea-son she had so few symptoms was that the early part of her test also showed very low blood sugar values, and she only rose to normal blood sugar levels for a brief period before she again went down to these very low values. She was "adapted" to low blood sugar—but not living very successfully with this adaptation. She cried when she was told that her diagnosis was hypo-glycemia. Her tears were those of relief, relief from the despair that had haunted her for many, many months. She knew that with this diagnosis something could be done, and she could return to her old self.

T. J. was the sort of man everybody admired. He had a position of authority, and he seemed competent in the position. He was good to know, and good to work with—a real leader. Recently, though, he had had a problem: alcohol. In his business a certain amount of drinking was almost routine, and not frowned upon. But now, at 57, he wasn't handling alcohol, it was starting to handle him. He still got to the office early, long before opening hours, and this was still his best time of day. He'd review yesterday's problems, read over the memos, and dictate his answers and conclusions. But his memos were beginning to look like those of a much older man; they rambled, they were fuzzy, and the conclusions were vague. He knew this as well as anyone and it disturbed him terribly. He'd watch the others come to work as had been his custom in the past. Some time between 9:30 and 10:00 he would have to leave the office. Everyone knew where he was going; there was only one bar in the neighborhood that opened early. He was becoming its steadiest customer. Did he have to have alcohol to work? It seemed to everyone he did. He'd come back thirty minutes to an hour later looking his old self. For a very short while he was his old self. He was clear, sharp and decisive—and his decisions were wise. But before very long, still early in the day, he would start to fall apart. The first drink or so in the morning had gotten him going, but it failed so quickly to keep him running that he became desperate. Now he wanted a drink, not to keep going but to get himself to the point where he couldn't remember.

Much too valuable a man to be put aside, he was counseled by his younger workers and his older associates, but with little success. No one really had a solution. He took a vacation for several weeks and came back with a tan. There really wasn't much other change; he still seemed to be going on the same schedule he was on when he left. More to placate the feelings of others than with any real hope that it would help him, he decided to have a physical examination. The exam was far from negative. His liver was in very bad shape, according to each of the several tests that were done for its function. His kidneys had some problems, too, though not so serious. He had a diabetic mother and there was some chance that he had diabetes too. In part because of this, he was given a glucose tolerance test. The results were not much different than in the case of Shirley M. His blood sugar values never rose very high, but stayed in the subnormally low range most of the time. Unlike Mrs. M. there were no tears when he was given his diagnosis. He had a bit more wrong with him than simple hypoglycemia, but all of it was correctable—if he could manage his alcohol problem. Undoubtedly, the alcohol problem had been caused by this hypoglycemia. He listened to the diagnosis—he already knew a fair amount about it, as was to be expected since he knew something about a vast assortment of things. In some ways he was a very easy patient to handle because he educated himself rapidly and easily on the theories and background of the disease. It became a challenge to show that you, as a physician, were as current and broadly informed as he was on this particular matter. Well aware of the poor showing he had been making in front of his employees, he seemed to make a miraculous recovery. In the mornings when he got to feeling badly, he didn't have to go downstairs to the bar any longer, instead he opened a small package of cheese that he kept in his desk and ate that. He felt neither the elation nor the confusion that the alcohol had caused, but he knew he was able to be himself once again. It wasn't quite as easy for him as it seemed to others. It was several months before he was able to cease having real cravings for a drink, and a year before he could allow himself safely to drink socially. As his hypoglycemia got better, he felt even worse. His blood sugar level would go down suddenly rather than stay down all the time. As a result of this, he would occasionally have sudden sweating, shaking spells which would drive him close to the edge of panic. Knowing what the problem was, though, he did not panic, although he did feel a certain dread of the next episode. That was a few years ago. Today he knows that years have been added to his life and to his effectiveness and he's quite happy to live within the few restrictions that are his lot.

Richard B. was the best salesman his company had ever seen. He was pleasant, comfortable, enthusiastic and a "real winner." At 34 he looked like the logical choice to be eventual sales manager. And everybody wanted to help him attain that goal. At the annual sales conference he was doing well with a speech on "Future Goals," when he suddenly had an attack. He was rushed to the hospital a desperately ill man. Since he was only partially conscious, there was little hope of obtaining much of his medical history. The diagnosis had to be clinical with some laboratory help. The story of his fall, as obtained from one of his associates, sounded like epilepsy. He had paused in the middle of a sentence, apparently aware of something about to go wrong. This is the "aura" of epilepsy. No one knew whether or not he had had epilepsy, although he had never had such an attack before as far as anyone knew. He had then fallen to the floor and his muscles had jerked back and forth in the characteristic tonus and clonus of grand mal seizure. He had no medication with him and one of his associates went back to look at his medicine chest and toilet kit to see if there was any that he carried with him. A few quick blood tests were done, and their results awaited. He was cold and clammy, which is not usual in epilepsy, and he had not soiled his clothing as many epileptics do.

The laboratory tests came back all normal except the blood sugar—that was 35mg%. He had hypoglycemia. Quick intravenous injections of glucose, a sugar solution, were started and Richard began to rally before half of the solution was in him. He was dazed and confused still, but he had reentered the world of consciousness.

The next day he was completely back to normal. The history of his disease was quite different from the histories of the other three patients. Richard had decided that this was a good time to lose weight, and he had gone on a fast. His fast wasn't complete. He had had an occasional alcoholic drink, but nothing more than this for approximately one week. He had lost twenty pounds, but had also lost his body's reserves. He was advised that his hypoglycemia would undoubtedly correct itself when he went back to eating his routine three meals per day. Still a somewhat scared young man, he took very little convincing on this idea.

Summary: All of these people had one simple thing wrong with them—too little sugar in the blood. Hypoglycemia doesn't often kill, but it has ruined many lives. The reasons that it occurs are still unclear, although people who are predisposed to diabetes are apt to have hypoglycemia before they develop their diabetes. It is most often seen in people who are overweight, and who slowly but steadily gain weight. Fatigue, either constant or in swings, is the most prominent part of this picture. Temporary relief from the fatigue, with sugar, is also part of the picture. It's not a fatal disorder, but it can be fatal to business and fatal to marriage if not treated properly.

Fortunately, the treatment is simple and largely dietary.

2

What Is Hypoglycemia?

To SAY that hypoglycemia is the opposite of diabetes is true, in the way that any oversimplification is true. The question then becomes: what is diabetes? A quick answer is that it is the failure of the body's insulin production or use. But that doesn't mean too much to most people. The best and real answer is that both disease conditions, hypoglycemia and diabetes, are related and they are related to the body's ability to use sugar effectively. Sugar refers to much more than that enjoyable sweet substance we find on the table and put in our cereal. Any carbohydrate we eat—fruits, vegetables and starches; breads, pastries and pasta—are turned into sugar by our body's machinery. The body's sugar is glucose. The various sugars we eat are sucrose, fructose and so on. No matter what they are, they are all changed into glucose by the body.

Dr. Rollin Woodyatt, one of the original diabetes specialists, compared these different kinds of sugar to money. Whether you have one hundred pennies, ten dimes, or four quarters, you always have one dollar. If you stay away from table sugar (sucrose), but eat too much fruit sugar (fructose), you still have eaten too much sugar. Of course, in table sugar all you get is sugar, but in eating fruits you get not only fruit sugar, but vitamins and minerals. But the important thing is sometimes the amount of sugar in a food. All nutritionists are aware that a balanced diet is necessary for health, but many people feel that if they eliminate one kind of sugar they have taken care of all of their sugar problems. This is not so.

Another difficulty many people get into is short-circuit logic. Sugar is sweet; therefore, anything with sugar in it must be sweet. Oranges are sweet, and they do have sugar in them. Lemons are sour, but they have twice as much sugar in them as do oranges! Bread and noodles don't seem particularly sweet, but their sugar value is high. One slice of bread equals about five full, heaping teaspoons of sugar. An ear of corn contains about twice as much sugar as a slice of bread! We have to have sugar in our diet because we use it for our major source of energy. As we have seen, people with too little sugar in their bloodstreams (hypoglycemia) can't be themselves, they can't function well. No one should attempt to go on a diet without any sugar in it. We've seen how difficult it would be to find a diet that had no sugar in it.

Do people get diabetes and hypoglycemia just because they don't eat the right things? No, but not eating the right things is certainly a partial contributory factor to both of these problems. Another important factor is one's inheritance. People with diabetes usually have a history of diabetes in the family: parent, aunt or uncle, or someone else among their relatives. This inheritance factor has been studied and is easily proven. Inheritance of hypoglycemia has not been as thoroughly studied, but most likely exists. Overweight is a forerunner of both diabetes and hypoglycemia. Hypoglycemia often develops into diabetes.

But diabetes is caused by a lack of a gland secretion in the body, a lack of insulin. At one time, not very long ago, this was thought to be the complete truth. Now we know it is at best a partial truth. Diabetics are treated by injections of insulin and their blood sugar controlled with this chemical. But most diabetics have normal or even high levels of insulin circulating in their bodies even as they continue to have the disease. Diabetes is not caused by a lack of insulin, but apparently by something within the body that interferes with the proper use of insulin. This is a problem not yet solved.

Hypoglycemia is a more recently defined disease, and has not had nearly the amount of research effort given it as has diabetes. Because of this, even less is known about the condition. Its cause is most uncertain. Dr. Franz Alexander, one of the first investigators of psychosomatic diseases, described hypoglycemia early as a disease that belonged in that category. His reasons for this we can already partially see. Emotional upsets, mental confusion, and lethargy are both mental and physical symptoms. More important, Dr. Alexander felt, was the fact that this disease seemed to be precipitated by psychic, emotional factors. Failure in love or in business, the death of a loved one, continued worry, were all factors he could find at the beginning of this disease. Another thing that argued in favor of its being a psychosomatic disease was the kind of drugs that treated it with a moderate degree of success. These were drugs which slowed down or inhibited the automatic nervous system. Atropine and its near relative belladonna were both used in this disease at one time because of their effectiveness.

More recently, Dr. Tintarra, founder of the Hypoglycemia Foundation, has gone a step further in this postulate. The pituitary gland, the body's main link between the brain and the endocrine system, may be the seat of the disturbance, he believes. His patients are treated with pituitary extracts, as well as with other drugs. Certainly drugs play an important, and at times even a necessary role in the treatment of hypoglycemia. We can be certain from the work of many investigators that the cornerstone of all treatments is dietary. This disease is no different from most others; early treatment means easier treatment, and usually more effective treatment. This is not a disease the body must continue to have, but one that can be reversed and the situation brought back to normal. I do not mean that this can be done without the help of a physician, but the major part of the accomplishment must be personal knowledge and adherence to the correct diet.

Not only is diet a matter of both cause and cure, it can also be a matter of diagnosis. By going on a test diet for a few days you may be able to decide for yourself whether your problem is hypoglycemia or something else. This isn't going to give you the full answer. The full answer most likely is going to come through one of those five-hour long blood sugar tests. But since most of us wish to avoid having hourly blood samples drawn for the better part of a day if we can, the dietary test is worthwhile in many instances.

So you take the tests, you pass them, and you still feel tired—do you forget the diet? No, this diet is based on nutritional common sense. Many times laboratory diagnoses cannot be made because of several factors. In the instance of this disorder, the diet you take immediately preceding the tests is as important as what is done the day of the test. This will be discussed in more detail in later chapters.

Is hypoglycemia a common condition? It's probably at least as common as is diabetes, and it is estimated that there are four million diabetics in the United States. Of this figure, about two million are known to have diabetes; the other half do not yet have the diagnosis made, though they have the disease. The number of people, and the frequency of both of these diseases, is apparently increasing. Most physicians feel that this is due to the general dietary habits that we all share. In this land of plenty we tend to eat plenty—far too much. Approximately 60 percent of the adult population is overweight, obese or fat, whatever you want to call it. They are more than ten pounds over their proper weight. This extra burden of fat, which is accumulated from too many calories from all our foods, places a strain on the body's mechanisms that handle the digestion and use of food. Some bodies are able to adapt to this strain and have no difficulty, others fail in this battle with too much weight, and these diseases develop as a result.

The dietary information that you will get in this book can help control your hypoglycemia, if that is the problem, or help you avoid it. Because it is a risk that too many people run with today's over-plentiful diets, education is seriously needed on matters of diet. As a physician told me many years ago, "If we all ate as diabetics must, we would all eat the right food."

3

Do I Have
Hypoglycemia?

DEFINING HYPOGLYCEMIA defines a symptom, not one specific disease entity. However, in this book we are referring to the most common cause of hypoglycemia, and treating it as a single disease. Hypoglycemia is a blood sugar that is lower than normal. In varying laboratory tests normal values for the sugar in the blood vary from 80 to 120 milligrams percent. That sounds simple and direct, but a person can have the symptoms and the upset of hypoglycemia while having blood sugars within this normal range.

There is more to it than the direct definition encompasses. A sudden drop of blood sugar down to a level of 80 milligrams percent can precipitate severe hypoglycemic symptoms in most people.

Its symptoms, as you already know, can be many and varied. Recurrent seizures and coma; mental aberrations and optical troubles, such as double vision, occur. Marked obesity is apt to be the eventual result of this disease if it is allowed to persist. Profound brain damage is, unfortunately, an anticipated result when the disease had progressed long enough.

Dr. Harry M. Salzer of the University of Cincinnati College of Medicine in Ohio points out three major divisions of illness that are related to hypoglycemia:

1. The major *psychiatric* symptoms of this syndrome are depression, insomnia, anxiety, irritability, lack of concentration, crying spells, phobias, forgetfulness, confusion and asocial and anti-social behavior and even suicidal tendencies.
2. The major *neurological* symptoms are headaches, dizziness, trembling, numbness, blurred vision, staggering, fainting or blackouts and muscular twitching.
3. The intensive somatic symptoms are exhaustion, fatigue, bloating, abdominal spasms, muscle and joint pains, backaches, muscle cramps, colitis and convulsions.

He also points out that hypoglycemia can mimic any neuro-psychiatric disorders. Patients with this syndrome have been incorrectly diagnosed as having such illnesses as schizophrenia, manic depressive psychosis and psychopathic personalities. Drs. Hoffmann and Abrahamson have demonstrated that hypoglycemia was present in many individuals with allergic disorders, peptic ulcers and rheumatic fever. In a book, *Good-Bye Allergies* by Judge Tom R. Blaine, with an introduction by Dr. Sam E. Roberts, connections were made between hay fever, asthma, migraine, hives or eczema and low blood sugar. Respiratory, gastro-intestinal and genito-urinary disorders also can often be traced to this underlying bodily disorder. Dr. Erwin Di Cyan states that, "physicians are increasingly getting to accept the idea that relative hypoglycemia not due to . . . tumors is a frequently met condition provided one keeps an open mind to recognize it."

Hypoglycemia may be the Great Imitator of today as another epidemic, syphilis, was a century ago. Because of its ability to mimic both psychosis and neurosis, some physicians recommend that no psychiatric diagnosis be made until proper tests are run to rule out the presence of hypoglycemia as the cause. Certainly any disorder that can cause this many upsets must deserve our respect.

It is rare that any symptoms occur before breakfast. A combination of fasting and muscular activity may cause the disease to be much more severe, with immediate symptoms occurring. This low blood sugar problem is encountered, also, in diabetics who are taking insulin or insulin-like drops in too great a dosage. Certainly other people also have this disorder because of too much insulin. These are upset or disturbed people who are able to acquire insulin and give it to themselves, even though they have no physical need for it. These are usually relatives of diabetics who exhibit recurrent hypoglycemic episodes, and usually vigorously deny the self-administration of insulin.

The body can also produce too much insulin, in the case of tumors of the pancreas or in conditions called the Zollinger-Ellison syndrome. This particular disorder is associated with severe stomach ulcers and other upsets. Other tumors, cancerous and benign, also cause this condition. Liver diseases occasionally give rise to the same upset. Other diseases that occasionally cause this are a low functioning thyroid gland (hypothyroidism), certain brain tumors, and failure of the adrenal gland (Addison's disease). These are not all the diseases that produce these symptoms, but they are the major ones.

The following list is complete although technical in nature. It is from a report in the *American Journal of Medicine* by J. W. Conn and H. S. Seltzer (left hand column). In the right hand column I have given the best popular translations of these names that I can:

1. Fasting Hypoglycemia (lowest blood sugar level in proportion to the duration of fasting):

Hepatogenic Hypoglycemia	Liver problems
Anterior Pituitary Insufficiency	Failure of the master endocrine gland
Adrenal Cortical Insufficiency	Failure of the adrenal gland
Central Nervous System Lesion	Brain and spinal nerve problems

| Fibromas Sarcomas | Cancer-like diseases |
| Severe Renal Glucosuria | Kidney unable to hold sugar |

2. Stimulative Hypoglycemia (normal levels of fasting blood sugar, but hypoglycemia two to four hours after the absorption of sugar):

Functional Hyperinsulinism	Too much insulin
Elementary Functional and Hyperinsulinism	Small-bowel disorders
Hyperinsulinism of Infancy	Rare childhood disease

3. Combined Fasting and Stimulative Hypoglycemia:

Organic Hyperinsulinism	Gland producing too much insulin
Idiopathic Spontaneous Hypoglycemia of Infancy	Disease of unknown cause.
Factitious Self-Administered Insulin, Without Diabetes	Disease of unknown cause.

The following charts illustrate various blood sugar curves and tell you more about hypoglycemia:

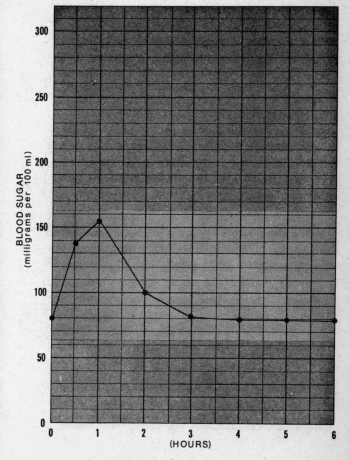

NORMAL BLOOD SUGAR
(Results of 6 hour test)

Chart 1: Normal Blood Sugar Curve

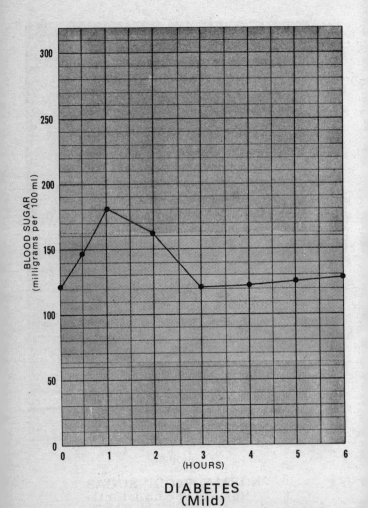

DIABETES
(Mild)

Chart 2: Diabetic Blood Sugar Curve—Mild

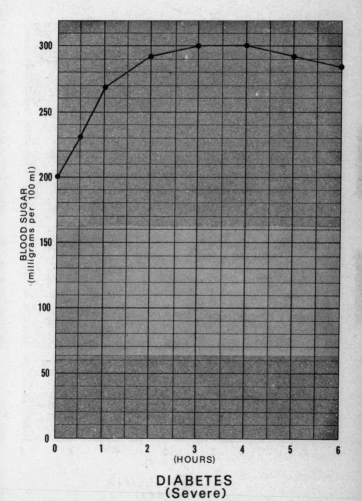

DIABETES
(Severe)
Chart 3: Diabetic Blood Sugar Curve—Severe

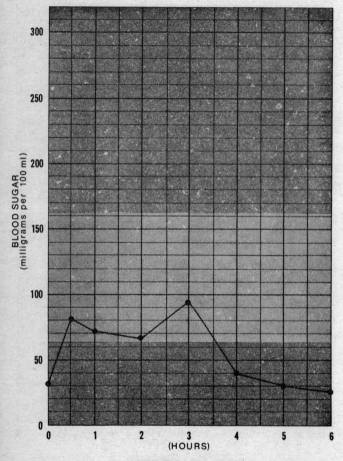

HYPOGLYCEMIA
(Severe)
Chart 4: Hypoglycemic—Fat Blood Sugar Curve

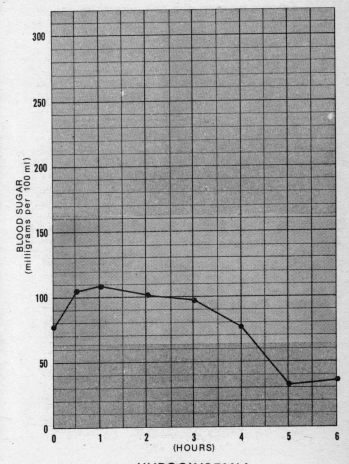

HYPOGLYCEMIA
(Common form)

Chart 6: Normal Glycemic with Hypoglycemic Ending

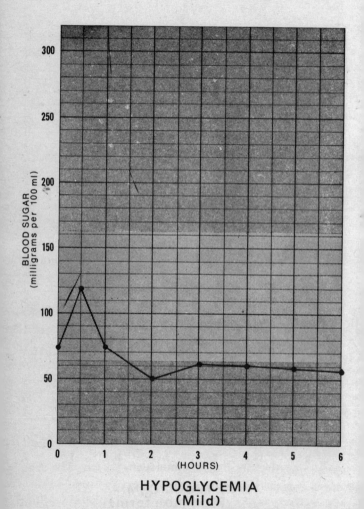

**HYPOGLYCEMIA
(Mild)**

Chart 5: Hypoglycemic at End of Period Curve

The signs of hypoglycemia are the laboratory findings of the blood sugar tests we have just gone over. The symptoms can be any of the symptoms we saw in the first four cases, or they can be other ones. The outstanding symptom is fatigue. Most commonly both mental and physical, though it can be only one or the other. Sudden sweating, varying from mild to an absolute drench, is a not too infrequent sign; the whole body may be involved, or it may just involve sudden excesses of perspiration in areas that ordinarily perspire anyway. These may be accompanied by chills, and usually the feeling of weakness grows greatest because the blood sugar is dropping rapidly in these sessions. This is the point where there is a real craving for food —some high energy food most likely. It might be candy, coffee and a sweet roll or some other pastry.

Many of these same symptoms are seen with another self-caused disorder, with an equally long name, hyperventilation. The fatigue isn't seen with overbreathing, which is what the word means, but the other symptoms we've just talked about are seen. You can find out if you are hyperventilating by checking your breathing. This sounds easier than it really is. Basically, you feel as if you're not getting enough air and you're trying to breathe faster and deeper than you usually do. And muscle cramps nearly always accompany this disease. Smoking a cigarette, though hardly recommended as a routine health procedure, will usually restore your breathing rhythm and stop hyperventilation. The diagnosis is made by having a person breathe in and out in an ordinary size paper bag. This returns carbon dioxide to the lungs and corrects the chemical imbalance that is produced by hyperventilation. This disease may also by psychosomatic, a sudden fright or a sudden feeling of despair or disgust frequently triggering the symptoms. Fatigue may help in precipitating the actual episode, but it is not part of the usual picture of a person suffering from overbreathing. Nor is weight gain and a craving for sweets part of the picture the way it is for hypoglycemia. The diagnosis is usually also the cure. Once a person knows he has a tendency to hyperventilate, and probably about ten per cent of us do, he also finds out what to do to correct this tendency. Hold your breath a minute, or 30 seconds, and everything straightens itself out.

There are other signs for hypoglycemia and I want to emphasize particularly that it's not necessarily a benign self-caused condition. Ninety-five percent of hypoglycemia is benign and self-caused, but the rest of the cases are due to some underlying illness—a condition that needs skillful and accurate medical attention.

Making the diagnosis at home can be quite accurate and true for a large percentage of people. But, are you a percentage? No, you are an individual. As an individual you must be diagnosed, and treatment begun, with a competent physician. You may feel sometimes that this is easier said than done. How do you know who is a competent physician for this? That's not as difficult a question for me as it is for you to answer. As a physician, I am somewhat able to evaluate other physicians. But, as a person living in the community, I need the services of other professional people, and I choose them the way I would recommend you choose a physician—personal reference. I take the word of one accountant as a reference to another accountant. And the word of one engineer for another. Each of us knows the competent men and women in our field, and once we know them we know we can rely on the judgment of other competent professionals in other fields.

Calling your local medical society is another excellent way of finding yourself a physician, but you must be able to help them by asking the right questions. If this is really the diagnosis, the man you wish to see is an endocrinologist. This is a man with "subspecialty" training. His basic training is that of an internist. Your community may not have an endocrinologist, but most likely will have an internist. There are nearly as many internists today as there are general practitioners, and this is why I refer you to them ahead of the G. P. There are, however, many general practitioners who have handled these cases with great acumen, and with very satisfactory results. There are men who have kept up with their education and not felt that everything they learned in medical school was sufficient for their lifetime. The other, "movie character," type of general practitioner is an extreme rarity today—and most likely not to be found. Certainly he would not be recommended to you by your medical society. There are general practitioners who have little interest in the diagnostic part of medicine and find that they are better and more skillful in other areas. If you visit one of them, I'm sure he will tell you as quickly as the medical society the name of a doctor with good training who could best serve your interest.

Now, you have the physician—you still must have

laboratory tests. We see all sorts of things in the paper about how awful laboratories are. All of us are human, some of us a lot more dedicated than others. Some laboratories do laborious jobs with joy, because they know they are serving sick people. Others don't even do routine jobs well because their interests lie elsewhere. Also, since they are human, accuracy of tests fades at 4:00 p.m. every day in every lab everywhere in the world. Do they all have hypoglycemia? I don't think so, but it is a common disorder. There is a way around this all-too-human ability to commit error. Automation has come to the laboratory, giving the same uniform, and in this instance delightfully inhuman, accuracy all day and all night. Not every laboratory in the country is automated, and probably even some of those that are have human errors in them. The odds against error seem much better, though, for two reasons. One, the automation itself is likely to be accurate. Secondly, these laboratories don't come cheap and anybody willing to make the financial investment is probably sufficiently dedicated to make sure they are run right. You have a part to play here, too, after you have found your physician, and after you have found the right laboratory. We'll talk about this later on.

4

How Serious Is It?

THERE ARE all degrees of illness possible with low blood sugar—mild, moderate, severe and fatal! And that's only the physical side. The mental upsets range from mild emotional problems through job loss, family fights, divorce and severe mental deterioration. That's not the whole story. Most people with this disease are in the situation of fumbling along. "Lives of quiet desperation" all too well sums up the problem that most hypoglycemics face. They are fat, not necessarily huge—though some are—but they are overweight and they have an uncontrollable appetite. There are times when they must eat, and this is a very true statement, they must eat or they may go into convulsion, and even die.

When does it start? That's a terribly important question. Did it start with an emotional shock? This is something you must sit and think about. Two days after your favorite parent died, did you start having trouble? Is it the same trouble you're having now? This is a ubiquitous disease, and not every psychic trauma need be the cause; there might be another reason. Pregnancy and the ensuing nursing, or lactation, can be a cause. But so can cancers and other tumors of various parts of the body cause it to start. A sudden severe infection might cause hypoglycemia, directly or indirectly. Sudden severe infections are one of the causes of thyroid gland failure. This results in low functioning, hypothyroidism, and in turn—hypoglycemia. (As an aside, the discovery of thyroid gland substance—at the turn of the century—did nearly as much to empty the psychiatric hospitals as the discovery of the tranquilizers has recently done.)

There are other serious conditions that occasionally cause this disease. We've gone over these before in all the detail that need be done. No need to go over them again. Their proper diagnosis requires far more than is possible to give in any book. A visit to your physician, and the use of the wide range of his facilities may be needed in order to get to the bottom of the problem.

CLUES

Liver Trouble: There are many signs of liver disease that a clinician knows to look for. Some of these early signs are apparent on the skin. Little red points on the skin with fine branching red lines going from them are one of the early signs. Because of their appearance they are called spider angiomas. When they are seen it's a distinct indication that something is most likely wrong with the liver. All of us are apt to get simple red points on our skin without these little red radiating lines coming from them and they are not the "spiders", but are thought to be changes of aging and are called *senile*. Dusky red palms, liver palms, are another sign of dysfunctions of this important organ.

Jaundice, characterized by a yellow color of the skin and membranes of the body, is undoubtedly the most dramatic sign of liver illness. It occurs because one of the functions of the liver is impaired: it is unable to get rid of bile as it should, and this bile accumulates in the tissues. The yellowness is caused by this accumulation of bile, and frequently a fierce itching also occurs because of this accumulation. Ascites, an accumulation of excess fluid in the abdomen, is seen frequently in far advanced liver disease. This accumulation of water occurs because of hardening of the liver—cirrhosis. The liver performs approximately 208 functions in the body, and life without it is not possible. There are many tests for the functions of the liver, and in the hands of a physician the troubles can usually be pinpointed and corrected.

Pituitary Problems: The pituitary is called the "master gland" of the body because it controls the functions of all the other endocrine glands. These include the thyroid, parathyroid, pancreas, adrenals, ovaries and testes. When a gland of this importance goes out of commission, even slightly, the results are going to be far reaching. This extremely tiny gland is located on a stalk at the base of the brain. Nerves from the brain apparently connect into it and in part control its function. Some have called it the "seat of the soul", certainly it is the seat of psychosomatic relations. When thought makes you sick or well, a great deal of its results are coming through the functioning of the pituitary.

One frequent example of this connection is seen when you are treating diabetic patients. It was my custom to place such patients in the hospital, bring them under control and educate them in their diet. Everything would go along well and their sugar output would become stabilized—until they were told it was time for them to leave the hospital and return to their private lives. This jolt would result, regularly, in their being out of control for two to three days; even though they were still in the hospital, still on their diets, and no other changes had occurred. We all need laboratories to know how to take care of patients with these disorders, but there was one statement they would make that would tell us they were getting better, regardless of what the tests might show that particular day. One way or another they would say, "I'm starting to think clearly", or, "I don't know what's been wrong with my thinking recently, but I see things differently now."

When the pituitary gland is severely upset, the effects are far reaching throughout the body. Weakness, wasting away, high blood pressure, disturbances in vision, diabetes, and kidney upsets may all occur. These symptoms are, fortunately, rare, and they are usually sufficient to bring their victims to a doctor.

Adrenal Gland Problems: The adrenal gland is probably next in rank to the pituitary in importance. These little triangles of tissue are located immediately on top of the kidneys. Their secretions come from the outer part of the gland, cortex; and the inner part, medulla. When we say we're full of adrenaline, we mean we're full of modular secretion. These secretions are for instant reactions in emergency situations—fight or flight responses. The more important secretions for daily living come from the cortex, which regulates water, salt, some sexual secretions, and many other functions. Tumors of this gland cause overproduction of the secretions and may result in the same problems that pituitary disorders can cause. Tuberculosis and other disorders can cause a wasting or atrophy of this gland, which is called Addison's disease. This results in a darkening or bronzing of the skin, diabetes, and a very profound weakness, a weakness far greater than that caused by hypoglycemia, and one that is relieved by the taking of large amounts of salt. It is only partially relieved by salt, but with present-day medicines it is possible to replace the secretions that this gland should be producing, and people now live with their adrenal glands removed.

Many serious diseases can cause hypoglycemia as a symptom; fortunately these are rare. There are other triggers for hypoglycemia that we haven't yet mentioned. Coffee, tea and alcohol are all on this list. Coffee and tea are stimulants and do their harm to us this way: although alcohol is a depressant, it is also a food substitute, and it is through its substitution and toxic effects that it causes hypoglycemic problems.

Coffee and tea both give us a "lift" because of the caffeine that they contain. This is a real result, not an imagined one, because giving straight caffeine causes the same effect. There is hardly anything in the world that doesn't have side effects, or effects other than the desired ones, and caffeine is no exception. In addition to the lift that we get, there is also a direct action on the body's sugar metabolism. The insulin production factory—the pancreas—is made to overwork by caffeine, and to this, in most coffee and tea drinkers, is added a sudden load of the sugar that's been added to either beverage. Nor should we regard coffee and tea as the only beverages that contain caffeine. All of the cola drinks have an amount of caffeine about equal to that of two cups of coffee. And they have as much or more sugar as well. These drinks all help with the immediate problem, but they are the real causes of the basic problem—hypoglycemia.

Since the common symptoms of this disorder are lack of energy, undue susceptibility to fatigue, disinclination to activity, headache, pains in the back, disturbed sleep, a drink of some caffeine-containing beverage often seems the right answer. It does mask the symptoms fairly well in many cases.

Alcohol: Other people don't find the necessary relief with caffeine and sugar, but need alcohol to mask their problem of hypoglycemia. Many physicians who have studied alcoholism feel that hypoglycemia may be the prime causative factor in many of those addicted to alcohol. In groups where tests have been made to see if alcoholics had hypoglycemia, the number of positive tests, indicating the disorder, have been extremely high, but alcohol does not have a simple cause and effect relationship of the other beverages. While it masks the symptoms, and gives temporary increased energy through direct metabolic action, it further lowers the body's stores of sugar and causes a worsening of the low blood sugar problems. Deaths have been reported from hypoglycemia in alcoholics.

Too often the presence of this disease without diagnosis is thought to be an indication of neurotic or neurasthenic symptoms. The sufferers are told to "snap out of it," or "get control of yourself." These added stresses do a great deal for the disease—they usually make it worse. The person who is suffering feels there must be a great deal of truth in the statements and wonders why he can't find his way out of the problem. So he drinks more coffee, more alcohol, and eats more raw sugar—and wonders why things get worse. There is an easy way out of this vicious circle, and fortunately it does not take too long to get rid of the worst of the problems. Usually a week or two after beginning the dietary treatment, the major mental and physical symptoms disappear. Not that that ends the disease—several months may be required before the treatment is fully effective—but by that time no treatment seems too severe because you're feeling your "old self" again.

5

The Diet Principles

THE DIET that you are going to use is high in protein and low in carbohydrates. The third dietary factor, fat, is usually found in the foods we eat as proteins, and it will be taken care of automatically with your protein intake. Your basic problem has been one of needing quick energy and getting it through intake of carbohydrate or alcohol. Since either of these dietary substances give quick energy, they seem to be the solution, and they are for the moment. Only for the moment—because it is this sudden rise of the energy level in our blood that has caused us to make too much insulin and keep a vicious circle going.

The object of the diet outlined in this book is to break up this vicious circle. There will be two types of diets listed, one will be a rigid diet to follow for only a short while, and the other a final diet to use as long as you need it.

In all diets, as in all of life, moderation is the key word. But for the short term diet it is not the key word. You must adhere to this diet very rigidly and not moderate it with your own desires at all. That's not too frightening when you realize you're going to feel totally different at the end of the first week than you have for a long while. You'll even feel different at the end of the first day than you have been feeling. Although we're talking about diet and foods, there are other factors we must consider. Coffee and tea are both stimulants, and they are great stimulants for the production of too much insulin. They must be avoided—almost totally at first. This can cause some distress because a person who is used to having a lot of caffeine-containing beverages, whether it be coffee, tea, or a caffeine-rich soft drink, is going to have withdrawal symptoms. The term "withdrawal symptoms" is usually reserved in medicine for withdrawal from some narcotic and presents a picture of extreme agony. That's not the case here, but it is going to be a period of discomfort. You might feel that the symptoms, often a headache and a feeling of weakness, could be relieved by taking aspirin or an APC tablet. Take an APC tablet that contains caffeine and it will put you right back where you started. A few aspirin tablets judiciously used can relieve most of the symptoms, but certainly should be used in moderation.

Alcohol is also going to have to be avoided. The "lift" that it gives you isn't going to be needed as you stay on the diet, but just like the coffee or cola drinker you're going to feel ill for the first day or two. Switching over to coffee is not going to be the solution any more than it is for the person who has been taking too much caffeine directly. One highball, not a cocktail, during the day can be permitted. Only a distilled liquor should be used, no wines, cocktails or beer are permissible in this part of the diet.

You have undoubtedly gotten into this shape by eating only two or three meals a day and having either sweets or alcohol in between these meals to get along. You are now going to be having about eight meals a day, which may sound rather amazing, if not impossible. When you go through these though, you're going to find they're rather small feedings with the object of keeping a small fire burning at all times rather than the occasional large blaze that has been causing the problem.

Do you smoke? Cigarettes are being shown to change our rate of metabolism and may have a profound effect. This would be particularly true if you were a heavy, more than two pack a day smoker. Stopping smoking is difficult—no one disagrees with that—but it is not impossible. It is probably unnecessary to stop smoking entirely, but a considerable reduction in smoking is usually necessary in this disorder. If you can cut down to ten cigarettes or less a day you will most likely get rid of the problems that cigarettes are causing you. Since approximately one million smokers a year are giving up cigarettes, it should not be regarded as an impossibility. There are various preparations on the market that are supposed to help one stop smoking—and some people have used them with good effect. Alcohol can have a much more profound effect on a person with hypoglycemia than with others. When you run out of sugar and use alcohol as your substitute fuel, you may overwhelm the body to the point of death. There have been several deaths reported recently because of this fatal combination: too little sugar, and alcohol. Of course, if you're on the diet you won't have this problem.

If you don't have these problems, but are only looking at the matter objectively, it may not seem as dreadful as it is. Not that any of us belittle death, but an illness of this kind might seem to be self-caused (and self-curable) to the person on the outside looking in. It's not that simple. The physical changes and the mental confusion do not disappear with the diagnosis, but need prolonged treatment and sympathetic understanding. Self-control is needed, on the part of the patient, but this becomes easier with each day of treatment.

Carbohydrate Deprivation Test

This is a one-week test diet to determine your body's response when all the ready fuel is taken out of your diet. This will show you how quickly and adequately the body can use its stored fat as a source of energy.

This is a test only, and should not be thought of as a permanent diet.

If you are going to find out whether or not you have hypoglycemia, this is the best way to do it. A glucose tolerance test is fancier and a little more difficult and considerably more painful than this diet test. Also, the blood sugar test indicates the momentary behavior of your blood at six or seven instances in a five- or six-hour time period. This diet test will tell you how you feel on a different diet, and at the end of the week it will have served to change your metabolism and make it possible for you to have a more accurate idea of the workings of your internal machinery than any other test will give you.

There's no particular time to go on this test—you can start right away, or you can wait until tomorrow, or even wait until the beginning of a week. Most dieters that I have talked to start at some definite time, and the weekend is often the easiest time to begin a diet. Saturday and Sunday can be managed much better by many people than can their week days. If they go into Monday with two days of diet consciousness behind them, they are much more able to continue the program than to start bright and early on that naturally difficult day—Monday. There is no particular place to go on your diet: you can be at home, on vacation, traveling abroad or taking care of an invalid relative at home. You are going to have to be able to have some control over the preparation of your foods or you may think you are on a diet and not actually be on it. Most cooks are going to put milk in scrambled eggs unless they're directly told not to. If you ask for "pan scrambled" it is less likely to have milk, but you had still better make certain before you eat it. If you avoid creamy salad dressings, such as roquefort, and stay strictly with vinegar, lemon and oil dressings, you should have no unknowns getting into your diet that way. Be a little specific about what goes into your food, and you can have a quick, accurate reading of what has been wrong with your diet in the past.

As you start to feel better on this diet, you may wonder how long you should stay on it. Stay on it at least a week before going on to a more liberal diet. It's best to use this diet for seven to ten days and then go on to the Harris diet, which is discussed in the next chapter. Remember, it's going to do you good—and that's the reason for your interest in it.

PERMITTED FOODS: Your diet is to be made up exclusively of foods on this list. Each item is to be pure and have no fillers or additives in it, no extra starch or sugar. The amounts you eat are up to you—this diet merely tells you *what* to eat.

Meats: All except offal (brain, liver, kidney, sweetbreads), sausages, cold cuts, meatballs or other meats with fillers.

Fish and Shellfish: All are allowed without exception.

Fowl: Any, but no dressing or stuffing.

Eggs: Cooked any way, but without milk added.

Desserts: Only "no calorie" jellos or plain unflavored gelatin.

Fats and Oils: Butter, vegetable oil, shortening and pure mayonnaise.

Condiments: Artificial sweeteners, salt, pepper,

lemon juice, mustard, horseradish, and sugar-free syrups. Any dry powdered spice may be used unless it has sugar added.

Beverages: Coffee substitutes, weak tea, low-calorie soft drinks without caffeine (Fresca, Like, special root beers, etc.), water, club soda, bullion and clear broth.

RESTRICTED FOODS (up to the quantity specified):

Cheese: Swiss, cheddar, blue, American (2 oz. per day). No cheese spreads, as cream cheese, fresh or cheese foods (Velveeta).

Salads: Leafy greens, kohlrabi, celery, cucumbers, peppers (3 oz.). You may have two such small salads a day with a salad dressing that may contain oil, vinegar, salt, dry spices, herbs, and anchovies.

Alcohol: 2 ounces.

SUGGESTED MENU:

Breakfast: Eggs, any style, or omelet—no milk. Ham, bacon, cheese or smoked fish—if desired. Beverage.

Lunch: Meat, seafood or fowl. Cheese or egg. Small green salad. Beverage.

Dinner: Seafood cocktails—no sauces. Meat, fowl or fish. Small green salad. Beverage.

You do not have to eat any of these meals. If you are not hungry you don't need to eat a particular meal. This diet contains no bread or flour-containing products, no fruits or juices, and no sugar-containing products or honey. Vegetables are eliminated, except in the salads. Dairy products and dairy substitutes are all eliminated: milk, skim milk, yogurt, soup and so forth.

The most common mistakes made in trying to stay on this diet are apt to be the use of the "diet products", such as candies, gum, fruits and breads. Many of these don't contain sugar, but sugar substitutes and other carbohydrates that the body uses the same as it does sugar. Many medications come in a syrup or candy form, such as cough medicine or laxatives, and should not be used during this diet. Many salad dressings contain sugar and also must be eliminated. Whole jello is quite rich in sugar and has to be avoided. The seasoned spice mixtures and salts have sugar in them and must be eliminated. Also, you cannot use breadings, sauces, ketchup or relish.

You will feel physically improved on this diet, almost certainly. The improvement itself is an indication of your need to alter your diet to get your health to return.

6

The Rigid Diet— Two-Week Plan

THIS DIET isn't to be used forever, but must be used for a week or two in order to give your body a chance to straighten out and act as it should. This is called the *Harris Diet* because it was first developed by S. Harris, M.D., the discoverer of hypoglycemia.

Although it's important to know what's in a diet, it's even more important in this diet to know what *is not* in it. The quick-energy foods, starches, caffeine and alcohol are the primary things to be avoided.

YOU MUST ABSOLUTELY AVOID:

A. Sugar, candy, cake, pie, pastries, sweet custards, puddings, ice cream, and all other sweets.

B. Potatoes, rice, grapes, raisins, plums, figs, dates and bananas.

C. Spaghetti, macaroni, and noodles.

D. Caffeine—ordinary coffee, tea and cola drinks, including the low-calorie cola drinks.

E. All wines, cocktails, beer and cordials.

The list may look a little discouraging because it contains all the goodies you are used to eating to give you the energy to get through the day. Remember, though, you have been literally whipping a tired organism—yourself—and you want to stop doing it. There are many things you can have in a sufficient number so that you are going to have an enjoyable diet. Let's go on to the list of things that are allowed and you can get over the blues the first list gave you.

YOU ARE ALLOWED:

A. Asparagus, broccoli, brussel sprouts, cabbage, cauliflower, carrots, celery, corn, cucumbers, eggplant, lima beans, onions, peas, radishes, sauerkraut, squash, stringbeans, turnips, tomatoes.

B. Apples, apricots, berries, grapefruit, melon, oranges, peaches, pears, pineapple, tangerines.

Fruits may be eaten either cooked or raw, but no sugar may be used either added or in canned fruits. If you have a canned fruit that is sugar-packed, rinsing it two times with water and then letting it stand overnight in water will remove the majority of the sugar and make it acceptable.

    C. Lettuce, mushrooms, and nuts may be taken as often as needed—they may be used as a snack at any time. But, one half an ounce—a small handful—of nuts: not more at any one time.

    D. Any unsweetened fruit or vegetable juice, except grape or prune juice may be taken.

    E. Weak tea, decaffeinated coffee, or coffee substitutes are acceptable beverages and sweetened with any of the sugar substitutes.

    F. Fruit desserts, unsweetened, low-calorie gelatin, are acceptable.

    G. Alcoholic and soft drinks, club soda, low-calorie ginger ale, whiskey or other distilled liquors, may be taken.

Now how does all of this turn into anything to eat? It's really not difficult—although it's going to seem a little bit unusual the first day or two. After that, if hypoglycemia is your problem, you're going to feel so much better you won't care to eat any other way.

DIET FOR THE FIRST TWO WEEKS

On Arising:

Medium orange or four ounces of juice or half grapefruit.

Breakfast:

Fruit or four ounces of juice, one egg—with or without two slices of ham or bacon, one slice only bread or toast with butter, beverage.

Two Hours After Breakfast:

Four ounces of juice.

Lunch:

Fish, cheese, meat or eggs, salad, large serving of lettuce, tomato or apple salad with mayonnaise or French dressing, vegetables if desired, only one slice of any bread or toast, dessert, beverage.

Three Hours After Lunch:

Four ounces of milk.

One Hour Before Dinner:

Four ounces of milk.

Dinner:

Soup if desired (not thickened), vegetable, liberal portion of meat, fish, or poultry, one slice of bread, dessert, beverage.

Two-Three Hours After Dinner:

Four ounces of milk.

Every Two Hours Until Bedtime:

Four ounces of milk or a small handful of nuts.

You can substitute small handfuls of nuts for any of the midmeal snacks. You may also use a one-ounce serving of cheese as a substitute, and these are frequently available in little foil-wrapped packages. If you are to have your one cocktail a day, it should be immediately before either lunch or dinner.

The object of this entire program is to give your body a level intake of energy, and it will do that. Will it make you fat? Probably it will do the reverse, at least at first. One of the ways to get fat has been shown to be the occasional intake of large meals. We will discuss this more later on. The late afternoon slowdown is going to disappear by the time you have a week on this diet. The first week is going to be difficult, but each day is going to be better than the day just passed, and you won't have too much trouble following the directions.

You must prepare yourself for this diet and make sure you have the proper mid-meal snacks available to you wherever you are. If you don't have them available and can't get them quickly, you're going to backslide immediately and be as badly off as before. When dinnertime rolled around you would have a ravenous appetite if you had not had the snack one hour before. This is probably the most important snack of all, but none are to be ignored or avoided.

Some physicians state that this diet should be followed for three months before going on to an easier diet. Only you can be the judge of the length of time to stay on this rigid diet. If you find that you are beginning to lose weight, from an obese level, certainly stay on this diet—it's doing you good. Also, if you find that skipping this diet for a day, say at the end of the second week, causes all your old symptoms to return, you have a definite indication that you must stay on it for a longer period of time. In most cases, two weeks is an adequate trial on this, and I have found that you can then go on to the more liberal diet.

Remember that our appetite is governed by our thoughts, but hunger is governed by the body. You won't be hungry at all on this diet—but you may have an appetite left over from habit. This habit will quickly readjust because you're going to be feeling so very much better. You're going to be thinking better, too. Our brain is extremely vulnerable to changes in its fuel supply and can't work well when the fuel isn't furnished in a regular fashion. I have never met a patient with a sugar problem, either diabetes mellitus or hypoglycemia, who did not notice personality changes. Frequently, their complaint on coming in for the first visit would be, "I don't feel myself, something in me has changed." On questioning, you would get a great deal of material about personality changes and upsets. In nearly every case, the first real feeling of satisfaction came when the patient found his old and stronger thought processes and emotions were coming back. You will find this too.

This is another version of the strict diet which you might prefer to use in your first weeks of testing. I would point out most strongly that if you have been having symptoms of low blood sugar and they are not corrected by this, you should hasten to your physician because you probably have an underlying condition which will require further diagnosis and treatment.

BREAKFAST

Cereal (hot or cold)	½ cup
Bacon	2 slices
Eggs	2
Fruit	1 serving
Cream	¼ cup

MID-MORNING

Egg	1
Milk	1 glass
Crackers	3 small

NOON MEAL

Fish, fowl or meat	4 ounces
Vegetables	2 servings
Bread	1 slice
Milk	1 glass
Butter	3 patties

MID-AFTERNOON

Milk	1 glass
Crackers	4 small
Cheese	1 ounce

EVENING MEAL

Meat, fish or fowl	4 ounces
Vegetables	2 servings
Potatoes	1 serving
Butter	5 patties
Oil—salad dressing	1 tbsp.

BEDTIME

Cheese	½ ounce
Crackers	4 small
Butter	1 patty

Although exercise is desirable and even necessary to keep in good health, it can be dangerous for a person with low blood sugar. Exercise should be taken regularly to be most effective and this is particularly important for you. Exercise should never be taken on an empty stomach, but shortly after a snack, when the body's reserves are higher and able to provide the necessary extra energy.

If you are going to indulge in extra and unusual exercise, you should fortify yourself with suitable foods. The foods that are best are bread or crackers, bananas, and cereals. Exercise isn't something we just take in a gymnasium or in a bowling hall. It can occur anywhere. Moving furniture or even a few heavy books can be sufficient exercise to be dangerous if you are not properly fortified beforehand.

Candy bars are the most universally available food and very easy to carry—but dangerous. They contain too much energy, too quickly available, and will get you right back into the problem you're working so hard to overcome. Little packets of crackers are easily available and stashing a few of these at spots where you are apt to do extra muscular work could be a very helpful thing. Cheese, particularly the pasteurized, foil-wrapped kind, is fairly durable and will survive outside of a refrigerator for varying periods of time, depending upon how cool the place is where it is stored, and this is a good energy source. The cheese may get pretty dry before you eat it, and lack some of the fine flavor that you would like, but it will be just as useful for your body.

7

The Final Diet

This is pretty close to a normal diet and is going to be easy to do. Don't think, though, that it's an easier way to find out whether or not hypoglycemia is the reason for your fatigue. If you haven't gone through the rigid diet and the modified diet you are not ready to take this one yet. Sure, it looks easy, and it is meant to be easy. But it's not suitable for diagnostic or curative purposes. It is a good, long term, good sense diet. But, it won't tell you whether or not you have hypoglycemia, and it's not the diet to start out on. After a few weeks of this diet you may be able to go back to a fully normal diet, with a group of three absolute and permanent modifications. These are:

1. Never, at any time, take an undue amount of sweets: candies, desserts, etc.
2. No caffeine—coffee, tea, colas.
3. A bedtime snack of one of the types described in this diet is a necessity each and every night.

BREAKFAST:

Fruit or juice—one serving
Cereal (dry or cooked) with milk or cream
Optional: one egg and two slices of ham or bacon
Bread or toast—one slice, heavily buttered
Beverage

LUNCH:

Meat, fish, cheese or eggs
Salad: lettuce, tomato, mixed greens; with mayonnaise
   or other oily dressing
Vegetables, buttered, if desired
Bread or Toast—one slice, much butter
Dessert—crackers and cheese
Beverage

MID-AFTERNOON:

Glass of milk, 8 ounces

DINNER:

Soup, if desired, but not thickened with flour!
Meat, fish or poultry—liberal portion
Vegetables—two servings
Potatoes—one serving. Rice, noodles, spaghetti or macaroni may be substituted with this meal.
Bread—one slice, if wanted
Dessert or crackers and cheese
Beverage

BEDTIME-SNACK:

Milk, crackers and cheese, sandwich, fruit

All vegetables and fruits are permissible. Fruit may be cooked, canned or raw, with or without cream—but no sugar. Canned fruits should be prepared without sugar, either by canning or by washing as previously described.

Lettuce, mushrooms and nuts may be taken as freely as desired now.

Juices—any unsweetened fruit or vegetable juice except grape juice and prune juice may be used.

Beverages—coffee substitutes and decaffeinated coffee or weak tea are permissible. If sweetening is needed, a sugar substitute, saccharin or Sucaryl (R) should be used instead of sugar.

Desserts—any fresh fruit, unsweetened gelatin, or low-calorie gelatin and low-calorie junket.

Drinks—club soda, dry ginger ale, low-calorie sodas.

AVOID ABSOLUTELY:

Whiskey and other *distilled* beverages.
Sugar, candy and other sweets.
Cake, pie, pastries.
Ice cream, ices, sweet custards and puddings.
Caffeine—regular coffee, strong tea, cola drinks.
Wines, cordials, cocktails, beer.

This is the basis of your diet, but you need to know more which is discussed in the next chapter.

8

Dietary Good Sense

YOU CAN eat all the foods on this diet, but select the wrong ones and you'll have problems. Not problems of starvation, but other problems of bad nutrition. This disease and many of the diseases we see today are due to a lack of sufficient knowledge about diet. Part of this is expressed on a legend you see on many vitamin bottles: "The need for . . . has not been established in human nutrition." This legend applies to vitamins, minerals and occasionally to other food factors. What the legend means is often interpreted as meaning a great deal more than it says. It does not say that the items are useless, but rather something else entirely. Either the scientific evidence for the usefulness of these dietary items has not yet been presented, or it has been presented and the scientists in charge have decided that the evidence was not sufficient. Now there are a lot of weird food supplements around, and there have been a lot more in the past, and in a way this has served as a protection to the customer. But at other times it has deterred people from taking vitamins that are useful and necessary.

The story of vitamin E is one of the most interesting stories I know on the subject. It was discovered by Dr. Cashmir Funk, the same man, who invented the word vitamin. At that time all vitamins were supposed to be protein, amine substances that were necessary to the *vital* functions of life. From vital amines he evolved the contraction "vitamine", which became our *vitamin.* For years this very necessary part of our nutrition had to wear the label: "The need for vitamin E in human nutrition is not established." For a long while all the scientific evidence was based on animal experimentation, and that cannot be directly brought to human needs. Rats and cattle became sterile, or could not produce offspring, when they were deprived of vitamin E. No such human experimentation was possible, and therefore no human need existed—according to some authorities.

Later on, certain anemias of childhood were shown to be directly due to the lack of vitamin E. Also, infants and children developed skin rashes when they were deprived of vitamin E by accidental experimenta tion. Enough other evidence has been accumulated to satisfy the scientists of the National Research Council that vitamin E is needed in human nutrition, and vitamin E no longer has to carry this label.

Amyloidosis, a hard substance that forms between the cells of the body, is one of the diseases that has been discovered in animals deprived of vitamin E. Several recent studies, from different research centers, have shown that amyloidosis, with the characteristic deposits, occurs in "older" people. As far as I know, no one has made a correlation between a lack of vitamin E and amyloidosis in humans. Nevertheless, our diet is short and scanty in its vitamin E supplies, and the presence of these unexplained lesions in older people might be a very useful clue to follow.

Aging, as we see it in older people, is not a normal or natural phenomenon. It is the result of a disease in almost all cases. The hardest diseases for many research workers to conceive of are those that are caused by an absence of something. They spend their lives, often quite successfully, searching for a positive factor —a virus, a germ, radiation or whatever—and they find it as the cause of one disease and another. This difficulty is not new: it's been present for a long while.

One of the other vitamin deficiencies, beriberi, was described along with its effective treatment, before the beginning of the twentieth century by a Dutch scientist, Dr. Eichmann. Its cause was the lack of a nutritional substance—vitamin B1—in the presence of the diet. A decade later, when the first great American textbook of medicine was being written by Sir William Osler, he stated that beriberi was most likely an infectious disease, even though Eichmann's work had been acclaimed throughout the world as being the first disease discovered to be due to vitamin deficiency. Years after this, low-income people in the southern United States, and even children in various orphanages, were given diets that were deficient in vitamin B1, and they developed beriberi.

We don't have every essential nutritional element clearly defined yet. The need for certain vitamin elements and certain minerals has "not yet been established for human nutrition." But our diet is not as good today, in many respects, as it was one hundred years ago. We eat a great deal of food that is not fresh, but is canned, frozen or preserved. Two important things happen in this process. Certain of the nutritional elements are lost or changed so as to be useless. The other, and probably more important change, is that things are added to our diet that no human ever ate until recent years. Let's stay with vitamin E. Although it is not the only important vitamin, we'll use it as an example. Fresh cereal grains have high vitamin E levels in them, and they may have many other important nutritional substances. The vitamin E and many of the other substances are removed in the process of milling, bleaching, freezing and otherwise preparing these foods for the market. If you buy a loaf of bread, many of these lost items are replaced because bread is "enriched" with a standard vitamin formula. But, if you buy any other bakery product, it does not have to be made of enriched flour but can be made of the flour from which these essential nutritional factors are still absent. There is an old song that states "the whiter the bread, the sooner you're dead." Various experimenters have produced all sorts of difficulties in animals fed on a non-enriched white bread diet. One of the first men to do this was a Swiss inventor who took the elements that were removed in the milling and processing of bread, and made them into a nutritional drink—Ovaltine. But that's not a panacea, there just aren't any panaceas.

Rushing off to the health food store may give you some nutritionally rich foods. It may also cost you a lot of money for "fad" foods that aren't going to do you a bit of good. Buying foods from organic farms, rather than from farms that use manufactured fertilizers, may give you a better quality of food. Part of this is due to the fact that such a farmer normally takes better care of his acreage, just because he is more interested in nutrition. But the fruits and vegetables that come from large commercial growers can be just as nutritionally adequate, if they are fresh. I only have one reservation on this matter. If the soil is over-fertilized with nitrogen, it is possible to get conditions where the vitamin A is literally washed out of the ground. This has been seen and reported in livestock grazing on freshly grown crops from over-nitrated soils. It has not been reported in humans, and most likely won't be because we don't get our cereals in uncooked forms as green grass, but after a great deal of processing has occurred.

We need fats and oils for good nutrition in wide variety. And they must be fresh: what's worse than rancid oil? Over the time of man's progress, many ways have been found to keep oils from becoming rancid. The Hunzias, who live in the Himalayas, are a very primitive people, but they live well beyond 100 years in good and vigorous health. They only grind the cereals and other grains and vegetable oils they need for each day. They don't try to preserve anything after it's manufactured, but only manufacture what they can eat for one day. They rely, quite wisely, on nature's own ways of keeping fats from becoming rancid when foods are left whole. The first "civilized" solution to prevent oils from going bad was cooling or refrigeration. This does help, but even at deep freeze temperatures, it's not perfect. Vitamin E is known to be lost as foods containing it are kept under deep refrigeration. It doesn't all disappear at any one time but rather seems to evaporate, bit by bit, as time goes along.

Hydrogenation has been one of the greatest advances in preventing rancidity. This is a chemical technique whereby fats are altered from soft fats to hard fats and can withstand a lot more exposure to light and heat than would be possible any other way. Until hydrogenation came along these fats did not exist and, for this reason, the people called them unnatural fats. Certainly there is no proof that the body can handle these fats adequately or build strong and healthy tissue from them. If these fats were only an addition to our diet, the chances of their harm would seem to be less than if they were, as they are, a total substitution for natural fats.

There are certain fats we must have in order to survive. These are called the essential fatty acids, and consist of three short unsaturated fats. Their names are linolenic, linolinic and arachodonic. We need surprisingly little of these fatty acids to survive, less than two percent of our daily fat intake. Most of our diets don't have that much of these essential fatty acids in them. Surprised? I certainly was when I first began research in this field. Research workers will tell you, quite correctly, that corn oil contains all of these essential fatty acids—in their purest state. It doesn't in the grocery store—it's hydrogenated. At least among the brands that I am familiar with. Safflower oil, which went through a period of having a rather bad name, does contain these essential fatty acids. Not every product that contains safflower oil is going to contain these unsaturated fatty acids, though, because some of these products are also hydrogenated.

There's more to nutrition with the essential fatty acids than just taking them—something else is needed too. There is in America one small group of well tested, closely regulated human guinea pigs who are fed adequate amounts of essential fatty acids. This group is the Astronauts. In spite of their diet, and general medical care, when they return from one of their flights they have a bad anemia. Why? Some research workers think, and I agree with them, that it's because they are not getting enough vitamin E. Vitamin E is nature's way of protecting oils against rancidity. It works for the Hunzias when they store their grains instead of milling them all at once the way we do. The anemia of these hearty men is the same type as seen in infants who have been deprived of vitamin E. Just having linolenic and linolinic acids isn't enough: you must have vitamin E at the same time if these oils are to be part of your nutrition and build good cells in your body. Otherwise, it seems that these oils may turn rancid in the process of digestion and be absolutely useless.

Laboratory Tests: If I'm short of vitamins, can't I find out by taking a test? I have surprised many physicians, who have called me in consultation, by telling them there aren't any generally useful laboratory tests for most of the vitamins. Vitamin C is an exception. Most clinical laboratories can run a test for this vitamin and tell the physician whether it is high, normal or low. There is also a test for vitamin B-12 which tells us how the body handles that vitamin. There are no other tests for the other vitamins generally available. There are a few being used in research hospitals, but these are not even well proven. Buy foods of good quality, cook them briefly and eat them quickly, is the best advice I can give you. The fresher your food and the higher quality it is, the better are your chances for good health.

A low dose or "maintenance" type of vitamin-mineral capsule once a day, with meals, is probably the best insurance you can have of nutritional adequacy. It's not a substitute for good food, but a very meaningful addition to today's foods.

9

Fatness and You

IF YOU are within five pounds of your normal weight, over or under, you most likely don't have hypoglycemia. Earlier, I mentioned the fact that many of these patients were heavy, some even very fat. But there are some, probably about five percent, who are distinctly underweight, and frequently appear prematurely old. The problem is the same for both the heavies and the skinnies—they can't draw upon their bodies' energy reserves as other people can. The thin people have an added disadvantage—they don't even have reserves to draw upon. And their problem is one that few people can understand. They can usually eat everything, and do eat lots of sugars, and don't gain any weight. Often they have a real battle on their hands just to keep at their minimum weights and avoid losing more. They get a lot of free advice from every heavyweight in the world, eat more of the wrong things, and find themselves with even more trouble as a result. If this is your problem, what can you do?

You can, and should, go on to the same diets outlined earlier in this book. These are not mysterious diets that will cause thin people to gain weight and heavy people to lose weight: they are diets to normalize your body functions. If you know how insulin acts in the body, you can then understand why these diets are successful. This chemical, insulin, does two things in our metabolism. It burns up sugar and converts it to energy, and it turns sugar into fat stores.

A thin person with hypoglycemia probably just doesn't have very much insulin at work. It is neither providing the energy nor building the fat stores. A heavy person, on the other hand, has lots of insulin at work. It is burning up the sugar too fast—and, at the same time, adding on extra pounds in weight. As you regulate your body through these diets, your insulin functions will return toward normal, and your weight, as well as your energy, will return to normal.

For a long while scientists felt that the only role of insulin was that of burning up sugar. They knew fat had something to do with this burning up of sugar, but not exactly what. Recent research has shown that these two factors operate: sugar and conversion of sugar to fat. This is very important, not only for people with hypoglycemia, but for diabetics. Not so long ago diabetes was regarded as being caused, in many cases, by overweight. Now it seems that it is the other way around. The underlying defect that upsets the body causes it to produce too much insulin. This production of too much insulin causes a weight change and the appearance of diabetes. Obviously, it can cause a weight change and the appearance of diabetes. Obviously, it can cause the appearance of hypoglycemia as well. Why one person develops one disease and another the other is still unknown. But this type of paradox is not unusual anywhere in biology.

If ten men, of equal age and in apparent equal health, are exposed to pneumonia, the odds are that three will get it, two others will get a very mild infection, and the other five will have no trouble at all! This is true not only with bacterial infections but with chemical poisons. If the same ten men drink wood alcohol, one or two will go blind for life, three to four will have visual disturbances and perhaps blindness for a week to a month. For unknown reasons the other individuals will be totally unaffected. Very interesting, you say, but how do I gain weight?

Diet is the largest part of the answer, but this is a psychosomatic disease, and an understanding of your probable emotional situation may help considerably in your final cure. A noted gastroenterologist, Dr. Sidney Portis, did a great deal of basic research in finding hypoglycemia. He tested and reported on 929 patients who had undergone glucose tolerance tests. In this group, 157 persons were defined as having *fatigue,* as distinct from the other 772 who had other symptoms.

Going into the histories of the 157 fatigue patients, Dr. Portis found common denominators in their life situations. They were all people who lacked interest in their work and had been forced into their particular ocupations by various circumstances. In every case there was something else that each of them would rather be doing. "Frustrated by their natural inclinations, these patients develop a protest reaction against their perfunctory activities." Doing their jobs with no zest, enthusiasm, or interest, the tone of the body's automatic nervous system most likely declines, and that may be the underlying reason for the endocrine failure and automatic nervous system dysfunction. This part of the nervous system is designed to adapt the internal bodily functions to their necessary tasks. Fear or rage tune a person up to fight to defend himself, or to flee—or otherwise meet some special emergency. This is generally agreed.

Dr. Portis believes, as do others who have studied this phenomenon, that "keen enthusiastic striving for a goal may have a similar, more prolonged, but less intensive tuning-up effect on the internal vegetative process. It is well known that perfunctory activity performed without emotional participation is more fatiguing than even strenuous activity performed with emotional participation. Clinical observations seem to indicate that fatigue and apathy developing during activity performed without interest are not merely subjective emotional states but are based on the lack of adaptation of the carbohydrate metabolism to the effort required from the organism."

This is still a very efficient working postulate of the

whole problem of the psychosomatic illness—body-brain conflict. Other physicians refer to this situation as the "Nutcracker" syndrome. Whether the individual is at home or at the office, he is often told that he is wrong and he shouldn't be doing things the way he is. The story of Tom A. is illustrative of this. He was a draftsman for a medium-sized company whose business had begun to fail. The company did not want to fire Tom, but they could no longer keep him employed as a draftsman. They kept him at his same salary, but reassigned him to porter and janitorial services in his old department. His salary was quite good, and his added insurance and pension benefits made it almost impossible for a man of his age to think of quitting and starting anew in a different plant. He got sick. He did his work, as he had to, but with no interest at all. His wife was not particularly understanding and berated him regularly for the fact that he had suffered this loss of status. He got sicker. He was diagnosed as having hypoglycemia, and put on therapy and diet. He improved somewhat, but more slowly than is usually the case. But his progress underwent a dramatic improvement when his company got a large order, and he was put back on his old job and his status returned. He stayed on the diet a while longer, as good sense would indicate. The sensitivity of his automatic nervous system to environmental changes indicated that this was his Achilles heel. Others might have stomach ulcers, heart attacks, or a host of other problems, and not be helped at all by the Harris diet.

In this case the diet helped him to "hold" and not slide back further. More important than the medical therapy was the social therapy of the job being returned to him. It's not always that easy, sometimes you have to go out and recast your own life. Circumstances may not work as well as Tom's did—just sitting in one place. You'll have the energy and the physical ability and the mental alertness to take control of your life situation if you're taking care of your body and preventing hypoglycemia.

The principles of diet are ones you should never abandon because, even years later, the symptoms can return if you do. You should have no sugar, either taken directly or in candies or in goodies from the bakery. Nor should you have any quickly absorbable starches: they amount to the same thing as sugar.

Your eating habits must continue to include a good breakfast, a mid-morning snack, lunch, another mid-afternoon snack and always a snack at bedtime. Cigarette smoking should be discontinued, or at least held down below ten cigarettes a day. Smoking before meals is forbidden by some of the experts in this area. The best time to begin to eliminate cigarettes is in the morning, before breakfast. Cigarettes smoked too early in the day do more to jam up the body's machinery than they do later on.

Correct your diet, correct your life situation, and you'll have so much pep and zest you won't mind these few restrictions. You will be so busy enjoying life you won't even notice them. They are part of the *new* YOU.

10

Other Elements in Good Nutrition

MOST OF us know the vitamins by initials, and some of us even have a fair idea of what some of the vitamins do. While the principal function of this chapter is to talk about lesser-known nutritional elements, a review of the better-known vitamins also seems in order. Before we do this, I feel that it is necessary to point out that, although a little vitamins are good, a lot are not necessarily better. The story of the Eskimos probably tells what problems vitamins can cause better than any other I know.

When the explorers first encountered Eskimos, they found that no matter how hungry the Eskimos were, they never ate the liver of the polar bear or of the seal. Many of the explorers regarded this as mere superstition; certainly the Eskimos could not give them any scientific answer for their fear of these foods. The explorers ate the livers—they got sick, some died. We now know that the richest source of vitamin D anywhere in the world is the liver of the polar bear. It is so rich in vitamin D it is poisonous. The seal liver has a goodly amount of this vitamin, too, and is equally poisonous. Nor is vitamin D the only vitamin that can cause death when taken in huge quantities; vitamin A has also caused fatalities.

Minor overdoses of vitamins won't kill anyone, but they can give a great deal of stomach and bowel distress when taken over a short period of time. When heavy doses of vitamins are taken over a long period of time, they have been known to cause arthritis and other disorders of the bones. Nature, when left undisturbed, leaves only small amounts of vitamins in foods. After all, the vitamins are as essential for the growth of other animals and plants as they are for man. The fact that we can go in and purchase vast quantities of concentrated vitamins at a relatively low cost doesn't mean that we have discovered some fountain of youth. But it is an excellent opportunity to make yourself sick.

Vitamin A is active in maintaining the normal epithelial tissue and for bodily growth. It prevents night blindness and undue dryness of the eyes—zerophthalmia.

p-Aminobenzoic Acid. This is an essential factor for the growth of most microbes.

Vitamin B. The original anti-beriberi agent. It is now known to be a mixture of chemicals and it is called the Vitamin-B complex.

Vitamin B-1. The anti-beriberi or anti-neuritic activity. It is also called thiamine.

Vitamin B-2. This stimulates growth and prevents certain eye, mouth and genital problems. It is also called riboflavin.

Vitamin B-3. Pellagra-preventive activity and a growth-promoting factor. Identical with pantothenic acid.

Vitamin B-4. In rats and chicks this prevents muscular weakness and may be a mixture of other vitamins.

Vitamin B-5. Probably the same as nicotinic acid.

Vitamin B-6. This promotes growth and prevents redness of the skin—acrodynia—anemia, and convulsions in animals. In monkeys a deficiency causes hardening of the arteries and dental caries. It is also termed pyritoxine and is given for prevention of nausea and vomiting in pregnancy.

Vitamin B-7, B-8, B-10, B-11. These are all probably mixtures of various other vitamins and are not needed in human nutrition.

Vitamin B-9. A name that was never used, since no vitamin was discovered for this designation.

Vitamin B-12. Prevents and treats pernicious anemia in man and promotes growth in animals. A similar compound is cyanocobalamin.

Biotin. This is a growth factor for microbes.

Vitamin C. Prevents scurvy. The effect was discovered 200 years before vitamins were known. It is also called ascorbic acid.

Choline. An essential compound that is used in the body's biochemical reaction.

Citrovorum Factor. This is a naturally-occurring compound, but seems to be unimportant.

Vitamin D. This prevents rickets. The most common compounds containing it are ergocalciferol and cholecalciferol.

Vitamin E. Prevents anemias in childhood, and perhaps in adult life. It is commonly found in tocopherols —alcohols that occur in nature, the three of which are respectively designated by the Greek initial letters alpha, beta and gamma. Many people feel that only Alpha Tocopherol is vitamin E, but this activity is present in all three of these naturally-occurring alcohols.

Vitamin F. Designates the activity of the essential fatty acids, especially as reflected in preventing hardening of the arteries in animals.

Folic Acid. Helps some anemias in man with a hematological response, and promotes growth in animals.

Vitamin K. Prevents hemorrhages due to hypoprothrombinemia. Also called anti-hemorrhagic vitamin and the prothrombin factor.

Lipoic Acid. This element is necessary for other vitamins to function (thiamine and coenzyme A).

Nicotinic Acid. The pellagra-preventing vitamin.

Nicotinamide. The pellagra-preventive factor.

Vitamin P. Believed to be necessary to reduce fragility of the capillary blood vessels. Its activity is related to citrin which is no longer considered to be a vitamin.

Pteroylmonoglutamic Acid. This is a compound necessary for the building of blood cells in man and stimulates growth in animals.

Vitamin U. A factor derived from cabbage which has been reported to cure stomach ulcers.

This list only tells you of the vitamins you need in nutrition; there are many other things you need as well. Certainly many minerals—zinc, magnesium, iron and many others—are needed for full health. The symptoms of many food deficiencies also include fatigue. Should you run out and buy one bottle of each of these vitamins? You would have to spend a lot of money if you bought each of the vitamins listed. You don't have to do that, but you do need to choose your foods well. If you're able to choose enough high-quality fresh foods at each meal, you probably don't even need the low dose "maintenance" vitamin once a day.

Most of us cannot be sure of the freshness of our foods all the time. Nor is freshness alone an absolute guarantee of high-quality foodstuffs. The methods of farming and cooking can do a great deal to change the quality of our foods. When oil is first put into a french-fryer, it contains a goodly amount of vitamin E. As this oil is used over and over again, the vitamin E is lost. A hard resinous substance forms on the side of the french-fryer which has to be taken out with an air hammer. This high heat method of cooking in oil certainly changes foods, and it probably makes chemicals that are "new" to human nutrition. How useful they are for our nature is an open question. Not so long ago french-fried items were a rare treat; today they are entirely too common. If we would eat them only occasionally there would be no harm likely to come from them. But if every lunch consists of french fries, and every mid-morning snack of that french-fried pastry, the doughnut, we may put foodstuffs into our system which it really cannot use.

When you buy a loaf of bread at the store, it is usually fresh and well wrapped in a plastic bag. As you open the bag, take a deep breath and notice the odor of the bread. Whether you keep your bread on a shelf, in a bread box or in the refrigerator, notice the odors which begin to come from your fresh bread in a day or two. The oils in the bread are becoming rancid—technically, they are peroxidizing, and losing their nutritional value. Some South American research workers feel that the eating of peroxides is one of the main causes of liver trouble. These peroxides are abnormal elements and our body can't turn out healthy tissues using rancid fats as its building blocks. In many instances, the best test of food is your own nose. Food that doesn't smell right undoubtedly isn't healthy to eat.

Food poisoning ordinarily means an acute and severe illness due to eating infected food. This is its dramatic and sometimes fatal form. We should be far more concerned with the slow and subtle food poisoning that occurs from regularly eating sub-standard, rancid or inadequate foods.

In their search for freshness, the food manufac-turers put many anti-oxidants into their food. This does keep the food from turning rancid, but what does it do to our body's systems? Our body must burn its food-stuffs and oxidize them in order to run effectively. Do these antioxidants interfere with this business of living? Or are they a slow, but efficient, food poisoning? The answers certainly aren't conclusive, but common sense seems to suggest that we do not depend for our whole nutritional program on prepared and preserved foods.

It's easy to stay on the diet recommended here and have proper nutrition. Hot cereals are all made of whole grain products and are adequate nutritionally. Other whole grain cereals include such things as Wheaties, Shredded Wheat, Grape Nuts and Total—this isn't a complete list, but it will give you a start. Dr. A. J. Carlson, the distinguished physiologist at the University of Chicago, said that there were two big lies we say every day in our life: "fresh eggs and whole wheat bread." Nevertheless, look around and you probably can find a source for fresh eggs. Real whole wheat bread is much more difficult to find and, perhaps surprisingly, the best place to find it is at the largest food chain stores in the U.S. They have no corner on the market, but seem to be more interested in making healthy foods than one might expect. When your diet calls for fruit, try to make it fresh fruit, not canned, or frozen, or dried. Not that each and every meal must have fresh fruit, but try to see that at least two-thirds of the fruit you eat is fresh.

It's far easier to obtain milk of high quality and cer-tain value than it is with most other foods. But the milk must be whole and it will usually contain, as it should, added vitamin D. Dry powdered skim milk does not have all the nutritional values that whole milk has, and is not for your diet. Dr. Hugh Sinclair feels that dried milk increases our body's demand for the essential fatty acids and that this increased demand is not apt to be well met with today's foods.

When you set out to buy crackers, you are going to have to be ready to read the fine print. The "table of contents" should state that enriched flour is present to be safest. If you have a cracker whose first ingredient listed is whole wheat, you should have a cracker that will provide good nutrition. On these "tables of contents" the manufacturers must state in order the ingredients by the relative percentages used in the product. More than a few products have to list their first ingredient as water! Should your cracker have salt on it? Probably not. You will find out later on the important role that salt can play in producing illnesses, and you should try to select a cracker that is not going to add to your problems. Any bread that is sold must be made from enriched flour—that is the law. If you have a preference for white over whole wheat—or would rather have rye bread than either, that's your choice. Just make sure it's fresh.

You are to cover your bread with butter, not with oleomargarine. When you are using butter you are using a natural product with proven nutritional value. The margarines are all made by hardening, hydrogenating, vegetable oils—and do not represent a fully natural product. The newer "soft" margarines represent a step towards better nutrition, but I have no way of knowing how big a step this is. It would be easy to find out if the manufacturers would label their oleo as to the sources of oils and the percentage that has been hardened. They don't have to; that's the law, too.

When you are buying your protein foods—meat, fish, or fowl—remember you are going to be eating a fairly small portion, and start to spend your money for quality rather than quantity. And don't buy a bargain in the butcher shop or fish store if it means it is something you must put away and refrigerate a very long time. Food values are going to disappear from these items if they are kept too long.

All the time make certain the cooking procedures used require the least heat, the shortest time and the smallest amount of water than can be reasonably used.

11

Other Ways to Gain Pep in Living

THE MARK of a civilized man is, unfortunately, often the mark of a physically and emotionally sick man. A civilized man is supposed to be rational and unemotional at all times, a planner for long-term goals. In 1897, William Osler described the traits which are characteristic of the highly "civilized" person: "A man who has risen early and late taken rest, who has eaten the bread of carefulness, striving for success in commercial, professional or political life."

Recently, Frances Dunbar, in her book, *Psychosomatic Diagnosis*, described the "consistently striving person of great control and persistence, a long-term planner; he is self-disciplined and presents the "need to get to the top."

Such a person is described similarly by Cleveland and Johnson (*Psychosomatic Medicine* 25:600, 1962) as a "person who presents himself as success-driven and independent . . . reveals in his responses great concern about behaving in a conventional manner, conforming to the accepted ethical norms and presenting to the world a controlled, cautious front." The main traits are competitiveness, desire for recognition, multiple activity, and sustained drive. Upward social and economic mobility with a striving toward higher status has also been noted in the studies done on these individuals. Those most likely to acquire illness show a greater measure of rational self-control than a comparison, healthy, group. Part of this, at least, stems from the fact that the patients were temperamentally unsuited to their very inhibited behavior.

This seems unfortunate because we arrive at an image of a man who tends to become a "solid citizen," committed to highly acceptable standards. The pillar of society means well and does well. Because of his concern for the socially-accepted norms and an eye to future achievement, he shows great control over his behavior, drives and impulses; his activities are guided rationally rather than emotionally. These are called "desirable" social qualities of the civilized man.

Salek Minc, of Perth, West Australia, calls him the

"typical Western man" and identifies him with several points:

1. He has a broad time perspective and a strong orientation to the future.
2. He seems to be self-directed and self-disciplined.
3. He is detached from strong desires for immediate gratification.
4. He selects activities for potential achievements, not for the pleasure of work itself.
5. Although in every choice there must be an emotional element, once this choice is made, further emotional influences are subordinated to rationally-patterned behavior.
6. He is reliable. When necessary, he drives himself to work through rational self-imposition.
7. He has a conscious awareness of responsibility and is rarely motivated by actual enthusiasm.

These are all part of the precept and practice of civilized society. They are imposed by one's self and by social and economic factors.

This picture is not drawn from the abstract—it represents you! Your problems are brought on by trying to be this "civilized" Western man. You can still be civilized, but healthier and enjoy life more if you will listen to the advice of these authorities—and make some changes in your thinking and living. Chapter Thirteen is going to give you some ways out of your dilemma. This book is meant to change you—for the better, the best. All of these changes are going to give you better physical and emotional health, and a far happier life.

Great prominence has been given to the role of *stress* in producing disease, and particularly in producing psychosomatic disease. We can see, here, what these stresses are, and how they have come to be. Emotional and chronic psychic stress seems to be caused by rational control of our "drive discharge", which prevents the *acting out* of the problems. The civilized pattern of human behavior leads to conflict and stress. Because of rational control, situations often occur where there is emotion without action, or action without emotion. Both of these are extremely unhealthy. During these periods of civilized behavior, the body manufactures various chemicals and hormones which are not properly utilized. These are called catecholamines or neurohormonal influences, and are produced in the nervous system. When they accumulate, it has been postulated, they exert toxic effects on various tissues—including the endocrine organ and the heart.

There are many ways that we produce excess catecholamines, even in everyday situations. Lennart Levi of Stockholm, has done considerable study on industrial stresses and the production of these chemicals. Specifically, he investigated the body's excess production of adrenaline and its related chemical compound, noradrenaline. Before he could undertake this study, he had to standardize the responses that the other activities of living cause in changing these chemical secretions. The other activites that change are body rhythms, body posture, intake of food and fluid, smoking, alcoholic and caffeine-containing beverages, drugs, physical activity, night rest before the experiment, and experimental stimuli and measurements. All of these factors he was able to standardize and, therefore, obtain valid results.

His first experiment was termed "Industrial Stress I" and involved a monotonous but attention-demanding task—the sorting of small, shiny steel balls of four very similar sizes in the presence of realistic and loud industrial noise. During the experiment there were variations in the intensity of illumination, a rush due to considerable lack of time, and critical observations from supervisors. This experimental situation dreadfully resembles the conditions of work to which millions of people in factories and workshops all over the world are being subjected every day during most of their lives. Two groups were studied this way. One group was clinically rated to have a high stress tolerance and the other a very low tolerance to stress, all within the range of normal variation. Both groups showed very similar excretion of these chemicals, far above the usual, normal range.

His next experiment was on the stress of office work. And, in this experiment, simple proof-reading with ordinary typewriter noise in the background was the task involved. Again, the subjects studied were divided into those with the high stress tolerance and those with the low stress tolerance, as rated clinically. Again, both groups excreted very similar amounts of the catecholamines. In spite of the fact that the stress here was much weaker than in the first experiment, some of the subjects reacted with great increases of their adrenaline secretions.

Pleasant and unpleasant emotional states without

any work involved were also studied. In the first of these experiments, entitled "Film Stress I", ten healthy male medical students were shown a program of thirty film clips disapproved of by the film censor board. The cuttings depicted murders, fights, torture, executions, and cruelty to animals. The primary aim was to study whether films as stimuli could activate the automatic nervous system in subjects as relatively sophisticated as medical students. The stimulus proved quite potent, as the adrenaline output went up significantly—about 70 percent over its normal value.

These same films were then shown to a group of healthy young soldiers and the same changes occured in their output of adrenaline and noradrenaline.

In the third experiment, "Film Stress III", twenty young women office workers were shown four entirely different film programs of 90 minutes each on four consecutive nights. The first program, produced by the Swedish National Railway Company, was composed of bland, natural scenery films. Despite the fact that this was their first experience with this experiment, the women reacted with a significant draught of adrenaline production during the film period, apparently reflecting their reported feelings of calmness induced by the film.

The next evening they were shown "Paths of Glory," a tragic and agitating film. During the showing, these young ladies had feelings of anger and excitement. And, at the same time, there was a significant rise in their adrenaline secretion.

On the third evening, they were shown "Charley's Aunt," an amusing comic film. There was, even here, a significant rise in production of adrenaline, reflecting, perhaps, the intensity of their feelings and not the quality of feelings that were being enjoyed.

On the fourth and final evening they were shown the film of the gruesome ghost story, "The Devil's Mask," by Mario Bava. During this film they screamed with fear and reported feelings of anxiety and despair. At this time, their excretions rose to very great heights. After this they were unexpectedly shown the highly dramatic and thrilling film of Robert Enrico, "An Occurrence at Owl Creek Bridge." Again, they reported feelings of apprehension, and their output of adrenaline increased to a degree, but not as much as before, since it was a very short film.

Love and eroticism are essential elements in most people's emotional lives. Their relationships to the nervous system have not been extensively studied, perhaps because these feelings are not easily produced in any controlled experiments. Thinking that it might be possible to deal with this problem by using suitable parts of high quality love films, Dr. Levi produced such a film.

This was composed of nine purely sensual love scenes taken from various films and chosen in such a way as to allow the subjects to identify themselves with the characters. This, the "Love Film Experiment," was shown to fifteen young women office workers. An attempt was made to isolate the love element, avoiding obvious elements of tragedy, comedy, aggressiveness, or anxiety. They reported emotional reactions of moderate intensity usually of a pleasant kind, and their adrenaline secretions remained normal, or nearly so.

Although these films were sensual, they did not show openly or realistically the shape or the function of human sex organs.

The films in the next experiment did openly and realistically portray the shape and function of the sex organs, and were considered unsuitable to show to the female office workers. For the "Sex Film Experiment," a sample of medical and physiotherapy students were chosen, about half males and half females. They were shown sexual films that had recently been confiscated by the legal authorities. Sexual arousal was the main emotion reported by both sexes, although the men rated themselves higher than did the women in the study period. This difference in reporting of the subjective reaction was paralleled by the difference in noradrenaline production, being higher in the males as a group. An even more pronounced difference between the sexes was seen in the adrenaline excretion, which increased by an average of 66 percent in the males. As an average, it remained unchanged in the females, although some of the individual excretion rates among the women were quite high.

The last experiment Dr. Levi reported was "Every Day Work Stress II," in which invoicing clerks were studied during four consecutive days when working at their usual job. Changes were made in their method of payment; though usually on a salary, they were put on extreme piece-wages for part of the experiment. No other changes in their work conditions were made. During the piece-work days, their output rose greatly —by 113 percent. However, this very high output of work was accomplished at the expense of considerable feelings of mental and physical discomfort. Half of the group stated they felt hurried, and all but two complained of fatigue, backache, pain in their shoulders or arms, during these piece-work days. During salaried days the physical complaints were entirely absent. Their subjective state of stress was paralleled objectively by increases in the adrenaline and noradrenaline production.

This has been one of the most detailed and significant studies on the effect of our daily emotions and duties on both our minds and bodies. During unusual situations of stress, the body responds with an extremely high output of chemicals. These chemicals can, in these high dosages, be toxic of themselves. Also, they whip the other organs and glands of the body into unnecessary and often harmful activity.

THE WAY OUT

If you've been in one of these "Nutcracker" situations you already know it's not healthy. But now you should know a lot better just how really difficult it is making your whole life. The ancient Greeks regarded a dilemma as a mythical bull, who could be brought to earth by grabbing one of its horns. That same advice is equally useful today. But, first, you must determine the horns of your dilemma.

Does your job match your abilities?

Are you progressing as you feel you deserve to in your job?

Is there another job that would be more fun?

Is there another job you could do better?

Are you trying to do two jobs?

How many of the demands made of you are unreasonable?

Is your financial situation improving or deteriorating?

Is your marriage enjoyable?

Does your spouse understand you?

Are you able to talk things over with your spouse?

Do you "have to do" things that you know are bad for you?

Do you smoke too much?

Do you drink too much?

Do you eat too much?

Do you weigh too much?

What else is it you would rather be doing? Whatever it is, you had better get to it. Attempting to live in a situation of continuous stress, despair, and fatigue is not living at all. It's the underlying reason you have hypoglycemia, and it cries out for immediate treatment on your part. The diet is going to help you think better and more clearly than you have been able to for quite a while. But, once you start thinking better, you must use this ability to solve the total problem.

12

Nutritional Dead Ends

Dɪᴇᴛ ʙᴏᴏᴋꜱ and cookbooks take up quite a respectable place in nearly any bookstore. Some of them are excellent and others are disastrous for you. A recently popular fad diet, the Zen Macrobiotic diet, has led to a certain number of deaths. The Zen diet is supposed to "purify" the body. This it does by restricting the intake of water, and permitting only a few grains to be eaten. Severe scurvy, from a lack of vitamin C, has been the cause of death in those who have followed this diet to its all too bitter end. This diet, like many, is given with a nearly religious fervor and following it is more a matter of conversion than good sense.

The bizarre and spectacular claims of nutritional pseudo-authorities seem much easier to believe than simple scientific statements. All degrees of food fadism exist. Specific foods with wonderful claims of permanent youth and vitality are probably as old as our habit of eating. One food enthusiast may tell of miraculous values of oysters or wheat germ or cottage cheese—and another may claim that oysters and ice cream are poisonous. Neither are right. Fish, for instance, is not a brain food, but it offers excellent general nutrition.

There's no specific reason that I've ever heard about for not eating fruit and milk at the same time. The idea that the milk will curdle is rather foolish, since it will curdle immediately in the stomach naturally as the first part of digestion.

Some people think that there are foods that should not be eaten together: milk and fish, milk and lobster, ice cream and rhubarb, buttermilk and cabbage—but all of that is nonsense. Yogurt was thought to be a life-prolonging food by some very excellent scientific research workers years ago. Yogurt is a good food, but its claims for special efficacy have long since been disproved.

There's a large variety of foods which have been called "special," from time to time—often said to prolong the human life span. For instance, beneficial results have been reported after the consumption of royal jelly, a secretion from bees. Royal jelly is a food particularly rich in certain amino acids, protein substances, and could help anybody who was not eating enough protein. That's hardly ever a problem in the United States today, however, as we tend to consume too much protein rather than too little. Honey does not contain protein to any significant degree—less than three- or four-tenths of one percent.

It was once commonly believed that eating a lot of red meat would cause high blood pressure. There is no scientific evidence that any of the proteins in red or white meats have any influence on blood pressure. Red meats usually contain more fat than white meats and, therefore, can produce obesity from an over-consumption of fat. Even lean meat, from which all visible fat has been trimmed, contains considerable amounts of fat.

That "wine is the milk of old age" is a belief that many people still hold. In old age wine can promote the appetite and provide a few readily available and easily digestible calories while making life more pleasant. The evils of too much alcohol, whether it comes from wine or another source, are too well known to need any discussion here.

Soybean products have been recommended by various authors, particularly because of the fact that they contain considerable amounts of lecithin. Some studies have shown that lecithin may be of value in preventing an accumulation of fat in the arteries and help prevent hardening of the arteries. Lecithin seems to act as an emulsifying agent, which means that it can bring other substances in dissolution. In doing this it may transport various fatty materials through the blood-stream and help them be better used.

The oldest continuous food fad probably is found

in the diets of athletes. The Greeks, when training for Olympic games, made sure that some of the contestants were fed a great deal of meat and fat—to insure that they would gain weight. Somehow, the full story of what this was all about has been misunderstood for thousands of years. The only athletes so fed were the wrestlers, and in their style of wrestling the heavy man had considerable advantage over the man who was of normal weight. The training table of any athlete should provide a balanced and sound diet, not one aimed at instant weight gain.

There are several reasons that food faddism is dangerous. It is a waste of money and, worse, fake diet cures often give a person a false sense of security and prevent his finding real physical problems. Some self-styled nutritionists recommend raw sugar in place of refined sugar, sea salt in place of regular table salt, and even lemon juice in place of vinegar. There's no objections to any of these foods, except for their price, but neither is there anything specially wonderful about them. Raw milk, milk that has not been pasteurized, has been advocated by those who believe that milk loses much value when it is pasteurized. About the only loss that occurs when milk is pasteurized is that of its vitamin C, which is only there in small and insignificant amounts anyway. Milk is not considered a source of vitamin C in any form. The protection that pasteurization gives us against various infections is tremendously important.

Raw vegetables have had their places in fads at various times. Whether strained, or put into a blender and turned into a liquid, none has shown any life-giving properties that aren't already present in the vegetables. Too much raw vegetables will upset some people's stomachs, although most of us should include some uncooked vegetables and salads in our regular eating habits. Some vegetables are much more palatable cooked than raw and are far more easily digested.

Celery juice doesn't cure indigestion or rheumatism, nor does carrot juice improve the complexion. Parsley juice may be a tonic in the same way that a drink of good cold water can be one. Garlic juice doesn't relieve high blood pressure—but enough garlic, and its attendant breath odors, will certainly relieve social pressure. No one will come close. Gall bladder upsets are no fun, but they're certainly not going to be improved by white radishes or lemon juice.

Black strap molasses is made from the very last step in processing sugar and, as such, it contains the dregs of all the processing that has gone on before. Just as a connoisseur will not drink the dregs of wine, I don't know why anyone should eat dregs or expect wonderful results if he does. Wheat germ is another food that has been accorded many miraculous properties by some people. It can be a source of essential fatty acids and of tocopherols—vitamin E—but so is whole wheat a good source. Whole wheat is usually a lot less expensive, and you are not apt to buy it rancid. Much of the wheat germ for sale in stores gives off a very strong odor when the jar is opened, and that odor is proof of its rancidity.

Yeast has been credited with correcting difficulties in the menopause, helping insomnia, preventing nervousness, correcting baldness, helping color return to the hair and skin, aiding digestion and preventing aging. I've probably missed some other claims, but this is already quite a list. Yeast is a rather low grade source of some of the vitamins of the B-complex group. If you eat a little it won't do you any harm; if you eat too much you'll start to find your stomach rising with gas, in the same manner as a loaf of bread.

Some of these food fads give extremely restricted diets, so poorly balanced that chronic fatigue or even actual illness may result. Fortunately, most people cannot stick to such restricted regimes over a long enough time to suffer permanent damage. Diet fads come and go with changing emphasis in medicine and nutrition. The pseudoscientist changes his lingo with the times. We all have general protection against mislabeling of products and fraudulent or misleading claims through the federal Food, Drug and Cosmetic Act, administered by the Food and Drug Administration. The only difficulty is that the law frequently moves slowly and that fad foods go on for a long time before effective action is taken against them. New fads crop up regularly and the promoters of them are very knowledgeable about methods of getting around the law. Your best protection is your own intelligent skepticism about extravagant and mysterious claims. In addition to this, book reviews and reliable journals, such as the *Journal of the American Medical Association, the Journal of the American Dietetic, Today's Health,* and *Science News Letter* and *Stay Young Newsletter.* These are likely to be the best guides in the choice of special diets and special diet books. Most of them can be consulted in your local library. Specific inquiries regarding questionable products or misleading advertising will be answered by the Bureau of Investigation of the American Medical Association, 535 North Dearborn Street, Chicago, Illinois 60610. Some offices of the Better Business Bureau and some chambers of commerce are also equipped to handle these inquiries.

13

What Can Exercise Do for You?

Y OU MAY be too tired to move, but we're now going to talk about exercise—the type you can and should be doing.

Exercise has gotten itself a very bad name. In recent years the President's Council on Physical Fitness and other groups have worked to improve its image but to many of us exercise still means calisthenics, gymnasiums, and poorly-trained instructors. Well, before you skip this chapter, let me assure you that that's not what we are talking about.

Much of today's fatigue comes from the sedentary life, with its lack of physical activity, which is part of today's mechanized society. Some of the causes of this fatigue we have seen in the chapter about the catecholamines—adrenal and noradrenalin. But all we discussed in that chapter was how these substances accumulate and rise to dangerously high levels in our body. We did not talk about how these chemicals could be put to good use, and burned off.

Only recently, in Hans Selye's book, *Pluricausal Cardiopathies,* has he demonstrated that exposure to cold and exercise are the best and most easily accessible means of preventing stress disease. Scientific evidence, based on many years of research in animal experimentation, show us that the idea of "toughening up" and of exercising may be old but is quite valid. The under-exercise disease—that we all suffer from—with its accumulation of endocrine poisons, can be turned to healthy endocrine organs by means of regular exercise.

The emotional disturbances that are caused by sedentary living are as correctable through exercise as are the physical deficits of our over-rested, over-fed, over-stimulated, over-protected lives. The program outlined here is one of minimal, but acceptable fitness. If you wish to add more to it—and I am sure you will —don't subtract this from your new living habits. Throughout Europe, many countries are sponsoring regular physical fitness programs for all of their "healthy inhabitants," because too many of them are "pre-sick" due to the current living habits we all have.

Training, by reducing the sympathetic tone, says Harold Mellerowica of Berlin, leads to considerably more effective heartbeats. The reduced sympathetic tone will also reduce the amount of endocrine secretions that are causing hypoglycemia. According to the investigations of Raab, the increased liberation of adrenalin and noradrenalin is reversed with muscle training.

Sedentary living causes a reduction in the maximal oxygen intake and the performance ability of the whole body. This condition is common in our sedentary lives and leads to many disorders, but is avoided by those who engage in regular physical activity. The Russians Letunov and Motylyanskyaya feel that one of the more important roles played by exercise is an augmentation of the vagal tone of the body which is shown by a slowing of the heart rate and a reduction of the blood pressure, in their cases. And also by a change in the corticosteroids in the body after a year of training. Sports installations, they point out, are common in the Soviet Union for systematic exercise training programs for middle-aged, elderly people. When they study in training period of two to five years, those who have been physically inactive show progressive improvement in their physiology. "These favorable changes are attributed to a shift in the central nervous system-mediated motor-visceral reflexes, especially to an increase of endocrine regulatory mechanisms. Universal prophylatic of this appears as one of the foremost tasks of modern medicine."

Avoidance of many of life's emotional situations

will, it is true, keep us from getting these great concentrations of chemicals in our bodies. But we don't want to avoid life's emotions—some of them are extremely pleasant. Emotions are a necessary part of mental health when properly used. These chemicals, which we discussed, are produced in our body for physical and muscular activity. If we engage in a sufficient amount of this activity we will help our body and our mind in every way. And we can do this without having to resort to complicated gymnastics.

Dr. Warren Guild, whom we have quoted already, tells us that 97 percent of the adult population in America is unfit today. This unfitness is not unique to America. In Sweden they have instituted a country-wide physical fitness program called the Four M's because of their concern over their physical unfitness, and its resultant diseases. Similar programs have existed for a longer while in West Germany and in Russia. Many of the other European countries have similar physical fitness programs. In Communist China there is currently an enforced revival of the Tai-Chi exercise program for every working man and woman in the country. One of the freedoms we have in our own country is the freedom to be physically unfit. It doesn't look like a very valuable freedom, but it also gives us the freedom to be physically fit in our own ways. Habitual physical activity causes the same kind of adrenalin overactivity that we have seen can be caused by emotional tensions. In the case of emotional tensions, it's probably due to exaggerated brain reflexes in the hypothalamic area. But in the case of physical inactivity it seems to be a deterioration of the systems that regulate the chemical flows in the nerves; this is termed the antiadrenergic counterregulation. Several studies have shown this factor in the United States, Canada and in Israel.

While lack of physical activity weakens the body's muscles and endocrine system by disuse, the overstimulation that is a part of our urbanized living keeps us in an almost constant alert reaction to which there is rarely a direct or vicarious outlet. This imbalance can be the cause of emotional disturbance, and, while combined with underexercise, gives us a pathological environment. This constant suppression of the "fight or flight" response is an additional stress and contributes to this disease. Hypoglycemia is far from the only disease that is caused by these situations. Muscle tension and poor posture combined produce "tension neck" and the common "tension headaches." Lack of exercise also means that we should eat far fewer calories than might be considered normal if we want to avoid overweight.

Progressive walking and jogging exercises should be the mainstay of most people's physical fitness programs. Various studies, particularly those done by Thomas Cureton of the University of Illinois, have shown that volley ball, golf, casual walking and weight lifting produce almost no improvement in fitness. Badminton and tennis three times a week were a little better. The Canadian Five-BX Program was shown to be relatively ineffective in two studies. Weekend activity did not improve individuals in contrast to those who took almost no exercise at all. Swimming, if done on a regular basis of pumping back and forth across the pool is an excellent exercise, and causes the use of a good many calories in its performance. Running is as good, or slightly better, than swimming for an effective exercise program.

Programs such as those that give only the "six seconds per day" isometric exercises, without the addition of endurance or isometric exercises, are practically useless. Rhythmic activities done daily, combined with an emphasis on adequate breathing, are most useful. These include swimming, walking, jogging, running, skating, and skiing.

Various reconditioning techniques have been tried to give fitness back to individuals who have ended regular physical training. About twenty years ago, Zatopek, the famed Czech endurance runner, developed a method of interval training using alternately short periods of running and resting. It has been used in patients recovering from heart surgery, neurocirculatory asthenia, healed heart attacks, and high blood pressure. In normal individuals it has been shown that work capacity can be doubled in twenty weeks of daily training. After forty weeks of training, the gains in work capacity became stable and could be maintained for a long while without further effort.

The first interval training session should begin with three work periods, usually running periods of 30 seconds each, alternated with a one-minute rest period. The number of work periods can be gradually increased to 30, of 30 seconds each, per session. It need not be that long to accomplish merely maximal benefits. The duration of the work period can be from 30 seconds to 1 minute long, with rest periods in between of equal length. The work periods per sessions, of six days a week, can be from five to ten minutes in duration. Running in place in one's own room is undoubtedly the most practical way to accomplish this interval training.

There are certain basic rules you have to follow in this, as in any, training program. You should run, swim or jog at a vigorous rate. Vigorous means enough for you to really feel it, and this is something you can check objectively. Take your pulse before you begin any activity. It's probably around 80 to 90—anything from 60 to 95 is within the normal range. If your resting pulse is lower or higher than this, you'd best check with your physician before you begin any exercise program.

Now, begin your exercise and do it for 30 seconds, fairly vigorously. Now check your pulse again. It should have risen from its previous level. Let's say you began with a pulse at rest of 84 beats per minute. It should now be 110 to 120 beats per minute if you're really trying. It shouldn't be over 150—that is the red line for your heart machine. If your health is moderately good, it will go down to normal and you can resume exercising the next day. After a strain like that you shouldn't try to exercise again the same day. Your heart has been too long underworked and the idea of a little extra load may have frightened it a bit. Once you have found the degree of exercise necessary to bring your pulse up toward 150 you have found your proper level of activity. I have met a few people who have been so extremely fit that they could not get their pulse above 150. To some of them this seemed a discouraging sign, although actually it's the sign of the healthiest heart possible.

Now, how healthy do you want to get? Five minutes a day which will give you five 30 second intervals of exercise, is a minimum program for fitness. Thirty minutes a day, half of that spent at rest, will give you nearly maximal fitness. A half hour every day may seem like a lot of time spent in physical activity, although for most of us in sedentary jobs it really should be the minimum. There are other benefits from this much physical activity. During this half hour you should burn up two hundred to three hundred calories. That's just as effective, if not more so, than subtracting that many calories from your diet—and it's going to help you get your weight under control.

But there are sports and other outdoor activities you like. Must you give them up? No, not at all. Keep any of them, or even increase your amount of participation in them. But don't feel that they substitute for the interval training program just outlined. They should supplement it but not be considered substitutes for it.

When our bodies have gone so long without exercise we tend to think of exercise as distasteful and annoying. We don't want to know how much we can do, but how little, and when we can skip it entirely. Well, there are times when if you have hypoglycemia, you should skip exercise. You shouldn't start out an exercise program at the same time that you're doing the first, rigid, diet. And you should stop exercise immediately if you begin to become shaky, excessively sweaty, or nervous. These are all signs that you're burning up more sugar than your body can replace quickly and that you need to stop exercising and have some orange juice.

Other than these particular instructions, though, you should exercise on a regular, daily basis. Ten to fifteen minutes should be your goal, although 30 minutes would be even better. When you do begin to exercise, five minutes of the interval training ought to be adequate for the first week. The second week go up to about 7 or 8 minutes, and by the end of the third week you should be doing ten minutes regularly. By that time, you're going to begin to enjoy the exercise for its own, direct, benefit. Be good to yourself—keep it up.

14

The Other Causes of Fatigue

As WE said earlier, if your weight is not within five pounds of normal, either over or under, the chances of your having hypoglycemia as the cause of your fatigue are great. But there are other causes of fatigue, and some of them quite common. Anemia probably heads the list of causes other than hypoglycemia, although it is not the only cause, and we will discuss some of the other common causes as well.

When anemia is the cause of fatigue, headache, dizziness, faintness, increased sensitivity to cold, roaring in the ears, black spots before the eyes, muscular weakness and irritability are all apt to be associated symptoms. Restlessness is an important symptom if the anemia is developing rapidly. In severe anemia drowsiness is frequent. The headache due to anemia may be extremely severe and resemble that caused by infections of the brain. With anemia, loss of appetite is quite frequent. Nausea, flatulence, abdominal discomfort, diarrhea, constipation, vomiting or abnormal appetite also occur. Sexual disturbances also occur; in women this is frequently a loss of menstruation—amenorrhea—and in men a loss of libido is frequent if the anemia is severe.

The skin frequently undergoes rather dramatic changes in anemias. The skin tone is lost and so is the elasticity of the skin. Thinning of the hair may occur and breakage of the hair is frequent. If the anemia is due to a lack of iron, the nails lose their luster, become brittle and are easily broken and may become concave instead of convex. Longitudinal ridges also form in the fingernails, and are practically diagnostic of an iron deficiency anemia.

The presence or absence of anemia is determined only by an examination of the blood. Its existence may be suspected and its degree can be estimated with fair accuracy by proper examination. The skin itself is not a reliable index of anemia. The membranes of the body, if not inflamed, may show pallor and help in the diagnosis; allergies will also cause the membranes to be pale.

The nails, of course, give several distinct signs of anemia. The palms of the hands also can reveal anemia through a lack of color. Color of the creases in the hand is particularly important. If they retain their red color after the other skin has become pale, the anemia is probably not too severe. If there is no color in these creases, the anemia is probably of great severity.

Several things can cause anemia, but the two most common conditions are a lack of sufficient iron in the diet and hemorrhoids. These latter are a frequent cause of blood loss that may be chronic and long continued. There are other causes of blood loss, such as ulcers, which also can cause severe anemia. In women, the nature of their menstrual periods, the amount of flow, the duration, and the frequency may also be causative. Exposure to poisons is an occasional and dramatic reason for anemia. These are not necessarily poisons acquired at work in heavy industry, but may be a result of hobbies, exposure to insecticides, or to the taking of harmful drugs. There are also inherited diseases which can cause anemia, and if a relative of yours has had an anemia or a removal of the spleen it could be very important to your own health history.

Iron deficiency anemia, which is the commonest anemia, can be corrected by taking any one of a number of useful medicines. Your pharmacist can recommend an appropriate one for you. If your diet is balanced and you have an adequate intake of foods rich in protein, vitamins and minerals, you should not have an iron deficiency anemia. If you have any other anemia, iron won't help it! That doesn't mean there is no help for other anemias, but you must visit your physician and let him determine the proper medication for you.

Weak spells, fainting and syncope can all be frightening symptons. This is particularly true if they are accompanied by passing out—a loss of consciousness. When not accompanied by a loss of consciousness, they are usually due to serious muscular diseases. Myasthenia gravis and familial periodic paralysis are the commonest causes of this type of weakness. These are diseases that are under continuous medical investigation and their treatment is undergoing continuous improvement.

The other types of faintness are usually all similar in their symptoms. They begin with a prodrome which warns the person of the impending faint. He begins to feel ill and becomes giddy. The floor seems to move and surrounding objects begin to sway or spin around. As this progresses, the senses become confused, there are spots before the eyes, and vision may dim and a ringing occur in the ears. Nausea and sometimes vomiting occur with these symptoms. If the person can lie down promptly the attack may be terminated without passing out. To the observer, the most notable thing is an ashen gray pallor of the face, and often the face and body are bathed in perspiration. This is followed by a loss of consciousness. The depth and duration of the unconsciousness varies. Sometimes the patient is not completely out; his senses are confused, but he may be able to hear the voices and see the blurred outlines of people about him.

In other cases, there is a complete coma and a total lack of awareness and ability to respond. This may last for seconds, or up to one half hour. Occasionally convulsions, that look like epilepsy but are not, occur also. More usually the person lies motionless and all the muscles are relaxed. It is frequently difficult or impossible to find the pulse and with the very shallow breathing and great pallor this may be mistaken for death. The strength of the pulse improves and color begins to return to the face very quickly. Breathing becomes both quicker and fuller. The eyelids flutter as consciousness is regained. Although mental alertness has returned, physical weakness remains, and if he gets up too quickly or too soon he may faint again. There are usually no after-effects, no headache or drowsiness, after these attacks.

There are many things that can cause these fainting spells, although the commonest is a failure of the circulation. This can be caused by mental factors—psychogenic, usually emotional, reactions to stressful situations. Prolonged standing, as seen in soldiers remaining at rigid attention, is also a cause. People with severe coughing fits may increase the pressure within their chest so much during a spasm that the blood is unable to return to the heart from the body. This causes a tussive syncope. Heart failure and shock also can cause this, as can acute injury to the heart muscle.

Hyperventilation can also be a cause, as we have discussed earlier. Small strokes, cerebral vascular disturbances, can be a cause, and the elderly have no particular patent on this as a cause. In younger people it may be due to a rupture of a congenitally defective blood vessel in the brain; in those over thirty it is more frequently due to a rupture in a hardened artery. High blood pressure can cause an irritation of the brain and this, in turn, can cause fainting.

This does not finish the list of things that can cause fatigue. There are many other diseases; most of them are called exotic by the medical profession. These include such things as berylliosis, brucellosis, and the carotid sinus syndrome. This list continues through histoplasmosis, hyperchloremic acidosis and hypokalemia. Hypothyroidism is in this list, and it is far from rare.

Hypothyroidism means that the thyroid gland is not putting out enough secretions into the body, and as a result the fires of the body are banked, rather than burning at their regular flame. This disease tends to run in geographic areas, although it can be found anywhere in the world. One of the great "goitre belts" is around the Great Lakes region of the United States; there is another severe "belt" in Switzerland and also one in Spain. All of these areas are short of iodine in their soil, and this is undoubtedly a major factor in the production of hypothyroidism. But if you live elsewhere, there is no particular guarantee that you don't have this disorder. The most characteristic symptom in differentiating this disorder from hypoglycemia is an intolerance to cold. People with this disorder are seen wearing overcoats in the middle of summer and untold clothing in the wintertime. In the wintertime it's so bad that they rarely stir out of the house, and usually need the room temperatures up at levels which make everyone else uncomfortably hot. Another item is that they eat very, very little and yet gain weight—this is all water or edema, myxedema in their case.

A low blood potassium, hypokalemia, is not an easy disorder to get: it usually takes intensive drug therapy to acquire. It does cause weakness, a weakness so profound that death can result. This is a rare condition, and one associated with other illnesses that are sure to bring the person to the doctor long before hypokalemia occurs. Unusual mental disorders, manic-depressive disorders, also can cause weakness in their depressive phase. There are a few other extremely rare diseases that cause weakness, but there is no need to go into them here.

15

Alcoholism

OUT OF our enormous population of two hundred million, we have at least three million alcoholics. As a disease it may not be as common as the cold, but it is an extremely common and frequent disorder. Most of us, fortunately, can enjoy the pleasures—and even the benefits—of alcohol without being alcoholics. But there are those who can't drink. Alcohol is not the only drug that our society uses and in one way or another approves. Caffeine, in the coffee, tea, and cola beverages, is certainly higher on the list of approved drugs—by society's standards—than is alcohol. The number that are taking sleeping tablets, remedies, and other medications undoubtedly exceeds the number of people who have lost themselves in alcohol.

It's very difficult for the man or woman who needs some quick energy because of his or her hypoglycemia not to feel the onus of needing a "quick one." But tastes differ, and the need for instant energy is solved by many through alcohol; a candy bar is the solution for others. The hypoglycemic doesn't need alcohol as an eye opener, not until much later in the game, but it's around 10:00 or 10:30 a.m. of a normal work day that this need for energy is first felt. If a drink is taken at this time, everyone in the office or plant knows that it's a problem! Yes, a problem, not necessarily related to alcohol, but to the body's needs for energy. If these people learn early enough that their problem is an overactive endocrine gland, not moral slippage, they may be set right without ever developing into alcohol-dependent persons. On the other hand, I am convinced that there are many alcoholics who would lose much of their craving if they would undertake the rigid and trial diets outlined here.

Alcohol has had a very difficult time acquiring a scientific rather than a moral status. In our country Prohibition still represents an era of history rather than the attempt to legislate morality that it was. This era, and its morality, is well expressed in the comments of William Graham Sumner, who said, "If a drunkard is in the gutter, that is where he belongs . . . until a policeman comes along and carries him off to jail."

Things have improved since those hysterical days,

and there is now a willingness to investigate alcoholism scientifically. Many of these investigations have led up different alleys, too many of them blind. Raymond Pearl, a distinguished statistician, felt that alcoholism was a vitamin deficiency problem. Not a vitamin deficiency in that ordinary amounts of vitamins were not present in the diet, but that these people needed far more than the normal amounts of vitamins for health. This theory still has some adherents, and many physicians of my acquaintance, and I myself continue to recommend high vitamins for a person suffering from this disorder. It isn't really proven, but desperate situations lead to desperate remedies, and this thinking applies to alcoholism.

Alcoholics Anonymous is a group of practical men who have always called on medical advice. Their practicality has shown their medical advisers many ways in which alcoholism could be overcome. Their twelve steps are a guide that is unbeatable. It certainly has resulted in many cures of this disorder that could not otherwise have been hoped for. The twelve steps are:

1. Admit that we are powerless over alcohol—and that our lives have become unmanageable.
2. Come to believe that a Power greater than ourselves can restore us to sanity.
3. Make a decision to turn our will and our lives over to the care of God *as we understand Him.*
4. Make a searching and fearless moral inventory of ourselves.
5. Admit to God, to ourselves, and to another human being the exact nature of our wrongs.

6. We're entirely ready to have God remove all these defects of character.
7. Humbly ask Him to remove our shortcomings.
8. Make a list of all persons we have harmed, and become willing to make amends to them all.
9. Make direct amends to such people whenever possible, except when to do so would injure them or others.
10. Continue to take a personal inventory and when we are wrong to promptly admit it.
11. Seek through prayer and meditation to improve our conscious contact with God *as we understand Him,* praying only for the knowledge of His will for us and the power to carry it out.
12. Having had a spiritual awakening by means of these Steps, we try to carry this message to alcoholics, and to practice these principles in all our affairs.

I have known many men and women who have been able to refrain from alcohol for a lengthy time even though they could only take the first step of these twelve. Part of the first step is the willingness to do without a drink for that day. If a person makes the first step daily for six months, he is probably over the worst of the craving.

There are those who detract from the works of Alcoholics Anonymous, saying that their definition of an alcoholic is too rigid. They state that an alcoholic is a person who was destined for the gutter and that there are no other definitions of alcoholism; that the alcoholic is a noticeably ineffective worker, frequently absent from his job, and with notable personality changes. There are alcoholics who are deeply committed to this drug and do not fulfill these definitions. Many who show up on the job each day, particularly on Mondays, and sit at their desks. They don't do much —and much of what they do is wrong—but they are physically present. At the end of the week, or at other appropriate times, they endorse their paychecks. Other than this they contribute very little to society in any way at all. They are clean and fresh, smelling of expensive colognes, but they are alcoholics. Although this is not a habit-forming drug, there certainly are those who have a craving for a drink. Why this craving? Alcohol is the quickest energy source known to man. Sugar comes in a poor second in the race to supply the body's cells with instant fuel. Sugar has to go through several chemical transformations that require many complicated chemical reactions before the body can use it. This is not the case with alcohol, it must provide immediate energy. So much so that no other food stores in the body can function until the alcohol that has just been consumed is worked out of the body in the form of energy expenditures. Who needs energy this instantly? Hypoglycemics!

Are you going to have a drinking problem? Several forms of self study have been suggested which can give you a clue as to whether or not you may. The Alcoholics Anonymous suggest that each day, for a week, you take two drinks. Never more, never less, and always the same alcoholic beverage. You're allowed to choose at the beginning of the week which beverage it shall be, but you must stay with it, no switching.

If you were able to do this two-drink test for a week in this fashion, the Alcoholics Anonymous will tell you that you do not have a problem with alcohol. However, if there are days you want to have none, you're just as likely to have a problem with alcohol as the person who finds there are days when he or she must have three or four. Saving up or overdoing are both signs of a psychochemical imbalance that is part of alcoholism.

The implied test of this book is the total abstinence from alcohol during the time that you are taking the trial diets. Either is going to give you a good indication of the answer to the question.

Charles H. Durfee, Ph.D., coined the term "problem drinker," and suggested that there were eight signs and symptoms that identified the personality. These are:

1. The lost night. Drawing a blank on one's activities for an evening is usually the first sign of the body's intolerance to alcohol. During the whole of the *night before* the drinker may have appeared intelligent, rational, and unaffected—but the next day he doesn't know what happened.

2. Extra drinks. The drinker suddenly finds that the drinks are too weak, served too infrequently, or a little extra is needed in the drink.

3. A sudden unwillingness to talk about liquor as a problem. This is usually accompanied by a readiness to accuse family and friends of imagined slights and wrongs.

4. Rationalization. Finding excuses for taking a drink. It usually goes to this point before there is a real

awareness on the part of associates and friends that alcohol is becoming a problem.

5. Unwillingness to attend social functions, meetings, or dinners where liquor is not served. The prospect of a drink is far more tempting than any aspect of a party or conference.

6. The hangover stage. The morning after is no longer a headache with marked fatigue; but acute muscular aches and pains, an excruciating headache, butterflies in the stomach and chest, with nausea and belching associated with terrible apprehensions, fears and feelings of guilt and shame. The only relief for this symptom is more alcohol. At this point drink becomes physically necessary. And acute hallucinations are not infrequent. Also, at this point a prolonged spree followed by sudden abstinence can result in the delirium tremens—the D.T.'s.

7. The appetite begins to fail, indicating gastro-intestinal disorders. Alcohol has become both food and drink by this time.

8. The final item consists of insomnia and irritability, and this is characteristic of the problem drinker.

Dr. Durfee concluded, "A person who finds himself with any one of these symptoms is in the gravest danger of becoming a true, compulsive drinker. Could this state be made perfectly and fully clear to him at the onset of any of these results of drinking, he might be saved from the messy life that awaits him if he continues to drink."

Alcoholism has been thought to be due to many factors, and different cases are probably due to different reasons.

One of the causes certainly is hypoglycemia. Frank E. had held positions of great responsibility in business, and still had a good job. When we first met, his income was less than half of what it had been five years before. At first, this seemed to be merely the result of life's bad breaks. But he didn't believe that it was just bad luck. He felt that there was something wrong with him, and he wanted me to find out what it was.

He appeared lean, healthy and vigorous. The results of the routine laboratory tests, about twenty-five in all, were within normal limits. His history, other than that of occasional drinking sprees, told us only one other item of interest—his father had died of diabetes. Because of this, he was given a glucose tolerance test and it showed a diabetic type of curve during its first three hours, the blood sugar levels running quite high. As it was continued, though, blood sugar fell to levels much lower than normal. He didn't feel cold or sweaty to the touch, but he told us that he'd really appreciate a shot of whiskey. He used all of his charm and sales techniques to explain to us why he should have this drink. He didn't get it.

We explained what his blood sugar test had showed us and told him about the diet he needed to get on. At the end of the test he had been given some orange juice and bread and felt much better, so much better that he had stopped trying to sell us on the idea that alcohol was the solution for his uneasy feelings. We were able to point this out to him and tell him this craving could be satisfied, far less dangerously, with food and a proper diet than it had been treated with drinking. Frank was already aware of some of the problems that alcohol was causing in his life, and he was partially willing to go on the diet.

He returned to the office a week later, and hardly any change was apparent in him. He told us that business pressures had been intense—one of the oldest excuses these people find—and that he hadn't been able to pay much attention to what he was eating. Even though we had a nice tidy diagnosis in hand, we didn't have an effective treatment plan working. As long as Frank's environment stayed the same, it appeared to me, his problems would stay the same. Frank had plenty of vacation time owed him by the company because he hadn't dared to take one. He knew he had been neglecting his work and felt that an absence of two or three weeks would be all that would be needed to lose his job. With Frank's permission, I called his boss and explained the urgency of an immediate vacation for Frank. His boss was well aware of Frank's many talents, and of his current problems that were preventing the use of these talents. Not only did he say that he would make certain that Frank had a vacation, he offered Frank the use of his vacation home, which considerably eased the financial strain of this period for Frank.

About three weeks after that Frank came back to my office and told me that he had managed to avoid alcohol completely for this entire period and felt much better. He asked what I thought about drinking now. Like many men in business, he felt that it was necessary to be a socially-adept drinker. I told Frank that I thought he could drink again, in time, but not right away. He was still a sick man and his body still couldn't handle its foods in a normal fashion. I believe that it takes six months to a year to correct this condition, but I told Frank that it would be a full year for him. I told him I didn't think that this was cautious, but just that he had too much to lose by trying for an earlier return. I suggested that he might think of joining the Alcoholics Anonymous or finding another outlet for his present mental state.

A few months later, I learned that Frank had left his job, and I wondered what had happened to his therapy. The president of his company, and a few of his associates, had set up a new business venture. They had selected Frank to run it, and both Frank and the new business were doing excellently. It hadn't required an awful lot of effort on Frank's part to stay with the diet once he got started on it. The results were all that anyone could have hoped for.

16

Sleep ...
Insomnia

RESEARCH INTO sleep has shown some surprising things about it, and particularly about insomnia. Sleep is a normal and active process of the body. It's not like passing out. We don't go to sleep because our brain is short of oxygen. It's a time of needed mental and physical repair and regeneration.

Sleep is caused by the activity of nervous structures in the midbrain which relax from their state of maintaining wakefulness. Because of the structure of the brain, these changes in the midbrain cause changes throughout the cerebral cortex, which is associated with the changes of consciousness. Scientists are certain that sleep is a normal, physiological interruption of our waking state.

Sleep research has been centered largely on the results obtained from the changes in the electrical activity in the brain, measured by the electroencephalogram. With this instrument four stages of sleep have been recognized. In the first stage the person becomes drowsy, and various parts of the tracing taken from the brain waves change. The basic waves seen in the brain are referred to as alpha and delta waves. In the first stage the alpha waves become regular with a rhythm of eight to ten per second.

In the second stage of sleep, delta waves appear and the frequency and amplitude of all of the waves increases. There is also formation of little spiked waves referred to as "spindles." In the third stage of sleep, spindles are no longer seen but the delta waves are very evident. In the fourth, and deepest stage, there continue to be more delta waves and a decrease of the alpha waves. By checking the ratio of alpha to delta one can determine whether a person is going toward sleep or awakening.

Water is probably the only thing in life that is more important than sleep; deprivation of either can result in death.

Experimental animals deprived of sleep will die in a few days, no matter how well they may be fed, watered and housed. Experiments on sleeplessness in humans have taken the form of enforced abstention from sleep for several days, with tests going on during the time. The longer these tests have gone on, the more bizarre has become the mental behavior of the subjects. Hallucinations, delusions, and feelings of persecution are all very common results of prolonged sleep deprivation. Fevers have also occurred. The most interesting fact is that a short rest, perhaps ten or twelve hours, after four or five sleepless days seems to be enough to restore the body to normal. Most of the sleep done at this time is the stage three sleep; very little stage one is needed to get the person who is that tired quickly to stage three. Nor is there much of the stage four, the very deep sleep, seen in this resting period. These findings first showed the importance of stage three sleep.

Rapid eye movements (REM), occurring under the closed eyelids, are seen only in stage three sleep. After much debate it has been fairly well agreed that this is associated with dreaming. This has been proven in several ways, most importantly by awakening the subjects, and asking them what went on immediately after REM was noticed. Other changes in the body are also observed both before and at the time of rapid eye movements. In males there is regularly an erection of the penis; in the female there is regularly a clitoral erection. The nature of the dreams is very inconstant—all types of dreams being reported—as is natural because this is the dreaming stage.

Stage four sleep, very deep sleep, is usually so deep as to be unremembered as sleep. The many stories that those with insomnia have told on them are undoubtedly related to this deep stage of sleeping. People who sleep through fires, smoke, sirens and gun shots are people deep in the fourth stage of sleep. When they awake they remember nothing about the happening because of the depth of their sleep.

Dr. Arthur Shapiro, of the Downstate Medical Center, prominent in sleep research, has done work with many people with insomnia. He has asked them all to keep a sheet of paper and a pencil by their bedside and write down anything that occurred to them during their "sleepless nights." He has gotten hundreds of sheets of blank paper, and only a very few with notes, over decades of this questioning. In the laboratory these people have shown a great deal of stage four sleep, very little stage three sleep, and would awake feeling as though they had not rested. This indicates that the prescription for a sound night's sleep might be the wrong thing for many people with insomnia.

Since too deep a sleep is not a restful sleep, you should do something to keep from falling this deeply asleep. One of the reasons for an extremely deep sleep is hypoglycemia, made worse by the lack of the bedtime snacks listed here. A large, starchy, sugary bedtime snack will run the blood sugar up momentarily and then allow it to drop far below the normal level. Great physical fatigue is supposed to cause heavy sleep but, obviously, it has not in those deprived of sleep for a long period of time. Physical unfitness, with a lack of regular activity, seems to be the cause of quite a bit of insomnia. Perhaps the most important thing to realize is that stage four sleep, even though unremembered in the morning, is still sleep and has given the body refreshment.

Some people are convinced of the absolute necessity of taking a certain ideal quality and quantity of sleep; they are obsessed with its importance, and are referred to as "sleep pedants." Because of their anxiety over sleep they become panic-stricken at night and remain truly awake because of it. They demonstrate the truth that peace of mind is an essential preliminary to sleep. They have an insomnia of quite a different nature from that of the insomniacs described before. Frequently people' in this latter group give insomnia as an excuse for all their inadequacies and failures in everyday living. These people want to sleep and worry about sleep loss, but their mental agitation opposes sleep.

Physicians have learned that there are some questions that just never get accurate answers. The amount of alcohol drunk, the number of cigarettes smoked, and the amount of sleep lost—all are apt to be over or understated to an extreme degree. Keep a clock by your bed and Dr. Shapiro's pencil and paper also. Make notes, if you are awake enough, as to the time you are awake and the time it takes you to become drowsy enough to fall asleep. If, after a week of this, you still haven't filled anything in on the paper you are undoubtedly a stage four sleeper. If you've run out of paper, because of the multitude of notes, your problem is undoubtedly that of anxiety, and you should take the steps needed to correct this situation.

Insomnia can be associated with trivial ailments or with conditions that jeopardize life. Neither the severity nor the persistence of this symptom indicates, necessarily, the seriousness of the underlying cause. Anyone deprived of the nightly restoration of energies supplied by sleep grows weary and his mental and physical vigor is impaired. You seem to lose your fund of reserve force. Your tolerance to pain, noise, and the countless irritations of everyday life seems to practically disappear. Your capacity for effective work is intimately related to the ability to sleep; in fact regular healthy sleep is the most reliable measure of sound health.

There are several types of physical disorders that may cause abnormal wakefulness besides hypoglycemia. These are fortunately less common, but you should be aware of them. Pain of the spine or nerves may be particularly troublesome at night. An upset stomach, whether due to mere indigestion or disease of organs of the digestive tract, often interrupts sleep. Stomach ulcers are almost punctual about the time they cause an awakening, 2:00 a.m., so regularly that some people can nearly set their clocks by the reoccurrence of this pain.

The "restless leg syndrome" affects men about ten time more often than it does women, and is probably caused by different factors in different individuals. Varicose veins, with their attendant slowing down of circulation, can be a cause. Other diseases that interfere with circulation in the legs, such as Berger's Disease, can also give this difficulty as an early warning sign of the slowing of blood flow through the legs. Simple muscular tiredness is only occasionally the cause of this, but can be relieved very nicely by taking two or three plain or buffered aspirin tablets at bedtime.

Another disorder affects women much more frequently than men and disturbs sleep—acroparesthesia. That long medical word describes the tingling numbness when we say a hand or a foot has "fallen asleep," or, "My hand feels like soda water." This may prevent falling asleep, or awaken the patient nightly with this distressing but not dangerous sensation. This is usually caused because the person is sleeping in an uncomfortable position without being aware of it and is applying pressure to nerves that are just under the skin. Nerves around the wrist, ulnar and radial, are both very superficial and it is easy for them to be placed under undue pressure. The peroneal nerve, in the leg, may also have undue pressure put on it where it is not well covered by muscle. When these nerves are squeezed, we get the familiar tingling, prickling "pins and needles" feeling in the fingers and the hands. Occasionally there are aching, burning pains, or tightness and other unpleasant sensations. Vigorous rubbing of the area restores normal sensation and usually not much else need be done.

When hypoglycemia is the cause of sleep disturbance, it is often easiest to tell by feeling your bed sheets. Are they damp? A severe drop in blood sugar, often called insulin shock, is going to result in a lot of cold perspiration. Another clue can be a sudden startled awakening associated with fear, and a lack of muscular strength. These are also symptoms of too little blood sugar. "Night sweats" are also seen in far advanced tuberculosis, and in other extreme fatigue conditions. If, in addition to the above symptoms, you have a cough, production of sputum—particularly if blood tinged—you had better go and be checked for tuberculosis right away. But if your weight is normal, or slowly going upward, it is far more likely that hypoglycemia is the problem. I hope it is, for it's a lot easier to treat, and you're going to have a lot better life as a result of the treatment.

Perfectly normal people fall asleep at different rates of speed. Some go to sleep almost immediately upon lying down, others may take ten to fifteen minutes before they are settled into a sufficiently drowsy state to go to sleep. This whole range is normal and should be of no concern to you. Sometimes it seems that most of the body is asleep but an occasional start occurs in an arm or a leg or even in the trunk. If this occurs repeatedly during the process of falling asleep, and is repeated night after night, it may be a matter of grave concern. It should not be. No one has yet figured out what the cause of these little muscular jerks is, and they often occur in the awakening state as well as when falling asleep. It may go away, or you may have to "live with it" but it has never harmed anyone physically. These nightly, independent muscle activities do cause a lot of mental distress because they seem so unusual. Once you are told they are not too unusual the mental distress should be relieved. This type of over-awareness of the body's actions occurs most frequently in people who are introspective and aware, very aware, of themselves and their environment. They are bright people, and usually quite charming, and successful. Dr. Walter Alvarez compares these persons to thoroughbred horses. They are not the slow, plodding dray horses, but the high spirited and nervous thoroughbreds. This is a dramatic way to state that it's all due to the way you are built, and it is not a disease.

You probably need seven or eight hours sleep a night

for good health. Recent research done in Philadelphia showed that many elderly men who had a multitude of minor complaints were cured by eight hours sleep per night. They were not given sedatives but just strict instructions to spend eight hours per night in bed trying to sleep. They did sleep satisfactorily, after one or two weeks of rearranging their previous schedules. Before this study began they had all been getting along on five to six hours sleep a night and complained of various muscular aches and pains, nervousness, indigestion, and a host of other things. A thorough physical examination had shown that they had no specific disorder— but they lacked sleep. Since they were men 50 years of age and older, they had all felt that the "old wives' tale" was true and they could get along well on less sleep. Since all their symptoms disappeared, and they have become brighter and more cheerful on the eight-hour-a-night sleep program, it seems evident to them that they have disproven this rumor.

You can't store up sleep; ten or eleven hours is not helpful, and if you need it it probably indicates there is something wrong with your thyroid gland. You should have that checked by your physician. You can skip sleep safely for one night and go on short sleep rations for two or three—but no longer with safety. Even one night's loss of sleep can make it very hazardous to drive a car or fly a plane. It can also make it very hazardous to execute a judgment in any complicated business or financial matter.

17

Good Days and Bad Days

OUR COMMON problem was well stated by Goethe in his diary March 26th, 1780: "I must consider more closely this cycle of good and bad days which I find coursing within myself. Passion, attachment, the urge to action, inventiveness, performance, order, all alternate and keep their orbit; cheerfulness, vigor, energy, flexibility and fatigue, serenity as well as desire. Nothing disturbs the cycle, for I lead a simple life, but I still must find the time and order in which I rotate."

We all know, from our own experience, how our

own lives fluctuate. Some days you can't do anything wrong, other days it's difficult to do anything right. Through research we know more and more about our biological rhythms and the way our physical and mental nature ebbs and flows. Much of this work has been done on the diurnal, circadian, twenty-four-hour rhythms. We can find reference to these twenty-four-hour rhythms long before the birth of the German poet. I once heard two physicians attest to man's universal low point as we rode across the desert in the early morning hours. One of them, who had practiced in the desert for many years, observed the beauties of the dawn. The other agreed partially, but quoted Homer, "Dawn's icy fingers, the harbinger of death." We all agreed with this ancient truth. Each of us, from widely varying experiences, had found out the truth of Homer's statement.

Dr. William Fliess, an associate and close friend of Sigmund Freud, studied other rhythms in our life which he termed biorhythms. He noted that a fever might "suddenly" come on a patient and just as "suddenly" disappear after a time. He made similar observations about respiratory diseases, and various nasal conditions. He was a specialist in the field of ear, nose and throat medicine. A study of case histories showed him that a periodic cycle governed the sudden flare-up and abating of various illnesses. He concluded that all changes taking place in the human organism were cyclic developments of a rhythmic nature. His discussions and correspondence about this concept we have on record, with his letters to Sigmund Freud as well as to Professor Albert Einstein and many other prominent scientists. Dr. Fliess felt there were two basic cycles in man's nature, a twenty-three day physical cycle and a twenty-eight day emotional cycle. To this, others have added a thirty-three day intellectual cycle.

During each of these cycles half of the time is spent on the "high" side of the cycle, the other on the "low" half of the cycle. Most people, scientists and others, agree from their inner being that there is some cyclic change, but wonder about the premises of biorhythm. The biorhythm cycles are dated from, and related to, the date of birth. This smacks strongly of astrology. Those interested in astrology say that predictions of future events, or statements about past facts, show the same relations in biorhythm as they do in astrology. Unfortunately, the scientific basis for astrology is not considered to be very sound by many in the scientific community. Anything that relates to astrology may, therefore, be held suspect for that reason if none other.

The date of birth is a very important one to the whole organism—because it is a very shocking one. Physically, the heart must change the channels in which the blood circulates immediately at the time of birth. The lungs, which have been inert throughout pregnancy, must assume functioning at once at this moment. Light, as a sensation, is perceived for the first time. These changes could "set" the biologic and biorhythmic clocks.

The phenomena of "imprinting" is known to be a very strong mental activity that occurs only around the time of birth. Little ducklings "imprint" the first moving object they see as their mother. Fortunately, most of the time they are right. In scientific conditions, though, they may see a human being first—and decide that this is "mother." Inanimate objects, if they move, can also be thought of as "mother" by the young ducklings. This imprinting shows that the hours after birth are strong mental stimuli as well as physical stimuli. This, again, could serve to validate the most basic premise of Fliess' theory. Other studies have been carried out directly on the biorhythm theory which appear to give further credibility to its claims. Retrospective forecasting, telling the time of a crisis after it has occurred, has been employed a great deal in this theory—and has been shown to be accurate. Crises occurred when the theory stated they should, and successes occurred when the theory stated that this would be a fact.

I first became aware of biorhythm in talking to a safety engineer at a scientific meeting. I mentioned, rather casually, that I was interested in biological rhythms or clocks. I opened a flood gate of information and was referred to Mr. George Thommen, the author of *Is This Your Day?*, the most significant book available in America on biorhythm. I was interested in this because of the story the engineer told me. He stated that he had reviewed over 6,000 accident cases and found that the "critical days" of biorhythm—which only account for 15 percent of the time—accounted for 85 percent of all accidents! Since accidents are the third or fourth cause of death in all age groups, their prevention has interested me for a long while. I wanted to learn more about this technique just for accident prevention.

Always, in scientific research, there are errors and accidents—and these are often more meaningful than the whole experiment. I learned of two "errors" in the prediction of biorhythm, and felt that they served to validate it even more. The first was the story of a man who had been "up" on physical, emotional and intellectual abilities—and yet had strained his back severely that same day. He was interviewed and asked why it was that he had hurt himself at this time. He was not told that he was supposed to be unusual, but was just interviewed about his accident. He pointed out a large bag of scrap metal that two men would usually pick up and carry from one point to another. That one day, he said, he felt so good he knew he could carry it all by himself. Obviously, he was not superman that day, but he felt that he was. It should have been a good day for him, but unfortunately he overdid his own abilities.

The other case was a man who had his accident one day after his "critical day," which of course is possible, but in doing a large study such as this each fact must be checked out thoroughly. After much questioning, it was found that this man was born in Hong Kong, on the other side of the International Date Line. When his birth date was corrected for his present locale, everything read our correctly on his chart. These both were exceptions to the accident study, but they were not exceptions to the biorhythm theory.

We are all familiar with the common twenty-eight day menstrual cycle of women. This is due to the rise and fall, the ebb and flow, of the female sex hormones in the body, particularly estrogen. Women commit crimes of violence, suicide, become emotionally ill and generally upset right around the time of their period—

a "critical" time according to the biorhythm theory. This periodic personality change in women has been written up in a recent article in the *Journal of the American Medical Society*, but it can be found in the writings of Hippocrates and Galen, two of the Greek fathers of medicine.

A group of English physicians recently decided to check the blood levels for estrogen in homosexual males. They found it was rather high, and it rose and fell in a cyclic fashion. This seemed like a thrilling new discovery, perhaps the answer to male homosexuality. However, they realized they had no control subjects, and decided to use themselves and check their own blood levels. They, too, had significant levels of this female sexual hormone that rose and fell in the cyclic fashion. This ended their research on this track for the cure of male homosexuality, but it did tell us something we did not know before about men's cyclic emotional changes. All physicians have been aware of the fact that males produce a fair amount of female sex hormones, and females produce a fair amount of male hormones, but this was the first evidence of a cyclic production of these hormones.

The female sex hormones, estrogen and progestrone, have been shown, in many cases, to be directly related to the emotions. The male sex hormone, androgen, has been shown to be related to physical and muscular strength. The twenty-eight-day female sex hormone cycle exactly matches the twenty-eight-day emotional cycle postulated by Dr. Fliess. Does androgen have a twenty-three-day cycle? If it does, and it has some cyclic variations, it would further the cause of the twenty-three-day physical cycle postulated by him. Research will be needed to prove this, but such research may be going on now. Androgen is not only needed for maleness and physical strength, but is also needed in all of the new production of body cells throughout the body. The decline of androgen may need to be corrected by giving extra amounts in tablets or injections. Its lack, both in men and in women, may be causative of some of the effects we now call aging.

The thirty-three-day intellectual cycle was postulated in 1939 by Hans Schwing, who wrote his dissertation, "Biorhythms and Their Technical Applications," at the Swiss Federal Institute of Technology in Zurich, Switzerland, where Dr. Albert Einstein also lectured and taught. The chemicals that are needed to make our brain work are only beginning to be investigated. The hallucinogenic drugs, LSD 25, marijuana and others, are of interest to physicians because, through their chemistry, we may understand brain chemistry better. Schwing observed that his patients had periods when they could apprehend their material very well, and other periods which were only suitable for review of matter already taught. He divided this into various time groups and finally arrived at the thirty-three-day cycle. If it is true, it undoubtedly has a sound biological basis, but far more research must be done to find it out.

What does this mean to you? If you have hypoglycemia, and have to go on a diet, it might mean a great deal. If you know your good days, no matter how you find them out, you know when you can diet effectively. If you know your bad days, you'll know when you will have to keep a rein on yourself in order to stay on the program. As you correct your own chemical imbalance, and correct your hypoglycemia, your good days will be a lot better and your bad days less difficult.

How do you find out *your* biorhythm? Introspection, looking into yourself, is probably the very best way. A simple awareness that you do have days that are good and days that are bad can be the beginning of a better self-understanding, and a better self-use. There are charts and calculators available for the calculation of one's future biorhythms. These are being used today by thousands of people, some for their own amusement, others to help validate this theory. This particular theory is not yet proven, although the overall concept of ups and downs is one we are all well aware of. Salesmen, executives and housewives all know that there are days when they can do anything, and other days when they shouldn't have gone about their appointed tasks. If you can predict, even with fair accuracy, when these days are, you can save yourself, and your friends and associates, a great deal of tribulation.

A great deal of interesting scientific research is being done in conjunction with the astronauts. Their biologic rhythms, particularly the twenty-four-hour or circadian schedules, are observed extremely closely. It is from such closely studied groups of men that we may hope to get a further answer on this subject of biorhythms. As longer journeys into space are undertaken, studies involving longer periods of time must be made. As these studies are made we will have further answers on this subject. We know, from several sources, that we are not 100 percent effective every day. Some days we are only 50 percent effective, and other days we seem to be better than 100 percent. If the biorhythm theory helps us understand this about ourselves, whether it is valid or not, it has given us another clue to the deep personal demand made on the cornerstones of one of the early Greek temples to health: KNOW THYSELF.

18

Our
Internal Ocean

WATER AND salt are tremendously important elements to our body, and receive too little attention in nutrition. Too little water or too much water causes death. The same is true of salt, although its effects are not so instant. There are few advertising campaigns to sell us on the virtues of water, and many for other liquids. Salt is also taken for granted, and since it's so cheap, frequently used with no regard for its effect.

The grammar school rule that eight glasses of water

a day were necessary for health still holds. Yet, it's ignored by many. Thirst is often assuaged with fluids that contain caffeine, sugar, alcohol, and other ingredients—rather than with plain water. Often the best solution—pun intended—is plain water. We get a lot of water in our food—some vegetables contain better than 90 percent water—and the processes of digestion and metabolism create water within our body. Nevertheless, we need to drink water, and 50 percent to 70 percent of our body's weight is made up of liquid. Since fat tissue is relatively free of water, a very heavy person may be composed of only 50 percent water.

Why do we need so much water? Our kidneys need about a quart of water a day in order to function, less than this can cause serious disease. Perspiration takes off better than another pint of water a day that must be replaced. Sweat, increased perspiration due to heat, is added to this water loss during times of exposure to heat. A certain amount of water is also used by the digestive tract. This water is not usually lost to the body, but it is in cases of diarrhea, vomiting or other upsets of the digestive tract.

If you find a great necessity to take a lot of coffee, or any other beverage, you might try substituting water. This can do a lot to smooth out your whole outlook and disposition if all you need is water. People with diabetes need a great deal of extra water; 16 to 32 glasses of water a day might be their need. Excess thirst, excess urination, excess appetite—coupled with weight loss—are the classic signs of diabetes mellitus. Like many classic symptoms these do not necessarily occur all at once to tell you that diabetes is the problem. But, if you have hypoglycemia now, it may progress to diabetes mellitus. The physicians that I have known who either had diabetes or have a family history of diabetes were always careful of their food intake, cautious of their liquid intake, and liberal in their use of water. It's no guaranteed way to avoid this progression, but it certainly is practical common sense.

When you talk about salt you mean table salt, sodium chloride. When I talk about salt I'm not too worried about the chloride part of it, but I am very concerned about the sodium part—the sodium ion. Sodium causes the body to hold extra water in its tissues. Getting rid of excess amounts of sodium requires a lot of extra work on the part of the kidney. When the body works, whether voluntary or involuntary, it burns up energy—and you feel tired. An over-liberal use of salt, which is one of the more common habits of our time, can be a direct cause of fatigue.

Dr. Walter Kriel of the University of Iowa states that we use eight to ten times as much salt in our daily food as is needed. He states, and he is certainly not alone, that all the salt we need is present in our foods as they are served—without any addition, in the kitchen, or at the table. If we eat meat, we get a very rich source of salt from it. We also get a certain amount of salt and other minerals in vegetables. This is not all the sodium, the dangerous ion, we get, we also get sodium in a lot of other foods and seasonings. When we add mono-*dium*glutamate we are adding the dangerous ion to our foods. Sodium benzoate is a favorite food preservative, and if you're eating a lot of preserved foods you're getting a definite amount of sodium from this source too.

In many parts of the country it's fashionable to "soften" the water we drink. When we soften water we remove some chemical ions, and add others. The easiest and cheapest ion to add in is sodium, and softened water is often rich in sodium. With softened water there may be another problem, too. Studies on the incidence of heart attacks have shown that there are more heart attacks in soft water areas than there are in hard water areas. The chemicals that are present in hard water may be helpful to our general nutrition. If they are, they certainly shouldn't be removed from our drinking water. Some people, when installing water softening, have made certain that they kept their drinking water supply out of the "soft water" circuit. People with a danger of heart failure can't tolerate salt, and have to be sure that they do not drink "softened" water because it can be a sufficient source of sodium to ruin their salt-free diets.

Every farm boy knows that you put out large cakes of salt-lick for animals on the farm. Not only do cows eat it, as they do need extra salt, but it is stolen by other animals. Does this mean that people are different from other animals? No, but our diet is different. None of the animals that need salt are meat eaters, just vegetable eaters. With our many sources of food, meat, poultry, and fish, we get a natural intake of salt that is quite adequate.

The over-salt diet that we do eat, according to Dr. W. Kriel, may be largely the cause of the high blood

ressure so frequently seen in our country. High blood
pressure is, as we all know, a serious disease. What we
don't know is what really causes it. Certainly one of the
better forms of therapy for high blood pressure is a low-
salt diet. This has been proven for over the last two
decades. Experimentally, animals can be fed high-
salt diets and will develop hypertension. Moderation
of our use of salt would seem to be good dietary sense
for this reason.

Dr. William Bortz of Philadelphia has shown that
moderate intake of salt, the amount present in our
usual diet, is sufficient to prevent weight loss. Specifically, his research involves people who are on a high-
carbohydrate and low-fat diet, which has been a recent popular reducing diet. The diet that he checked
provided only 600 calories a day and would seem certain, because of these low calories, to assure weight
loss in anyone. This is no more important a finding than
the high blood pressure finding, but may have more
immediate meaning to many of us. High blood pressure and obesity are diseases that are frequently found
together. Even more important, weight reduction frequently helps control, or even cure, high blood pressure.

If you've been using very little added salt in your
foods, changing your habits is going to work no hard-
ship. You should check to find out how much salt is
added to your foods before it is served on the table. If
you like the flavor of salt and use a great deal of it on
your food you may feel that this is going to be a dreadful change. It need not be. There are salt substitutes
just as there are sugar substitutes, and their safety has

not been questioned. Some salt substitutes can only be put on the food after cooking, and others can be used in cooking. You can get this information from the labels. Occasionally, a salt substitute that can be used in cooking is going to be more useful because some food preparations require salt. This does not mean you must use the salt substitute each time you use salt in the kitchen; only when the salt is going to be absorbed in the food should the substitute be used.

I have had a lot of patients who came to me with stories of irritated and upset stomachs after eating at particular restaurants. My investigation showed that these restaurants used a great deal of meat tenderizer in producing their "prime" steaks and beef. Meat tenderizer, if properly used, and the directions followed should be of very little hazard. However, the directions are often ignored and the net result is that there is tenderizer left in the meat when it is served. This tenderizer is a chemical, of one sort or another, with only one mission in life—to break down meat fibers. It doesn't differentiate between the beef fiber that it is supposed to tenderize and the fibers of one's stomach if it gets in there. Be careful of meat tenderizers and certainly use them strictly according to their directions.

Sugar substitutes are made of either one of two chemicals, saccharin or cyclamate. We see a great deal about both of these being investigated by the Food and Drug Administration for their safety. Saccharin was invented in Germany during the time of World War I and certainly has a long history of use. Cyclamate is much newer and had more scientific investigation into its potential for danger before it was ever put on the market. I do not feel that the likelihood of anything being found dangerous in either of these agents is very great. But, certainly, it would be foolish to second guess research that is now being carried out. We should not need all of our food heavily sweetened any more than we need it heavily salted. As always, the answer to flavors in diets should be the general answer for the good life—moderation.

19

Recapture the Zest for Living

IF YOU misuse your muscles, you're a
to know about it quickly. You're going to feel i
mediate pain. If you under use them they will atrop
and leave you without strength. When the endocri
system is overworked or underworked, its problems a
equally great, but they don't show up in the same d
matic ways. Hypoglycemia is a disorder related to
strain on the endocrine glands. This strain is usua
dietary and environmental—emotions, situations a
fatigue. If you have hypoglycemia, and want to get

of its grasp, we have shown you the program that will do this successfully.

The first day's diet isn't going to cause you to have an absolutely new life, but you will begin to feel better. Don't go on a day and off a day; you're learning nothing and not helping yourself. Make up your mind you're going to be on the diet, the strict one, for a full seven-day period. Give it, and yourself, a fair chance. At the end of the week, your hypoglycemia will be less, and the symptoms will be lessened. You may progress to the other diets as your pep and strength improve. You should realize, though, that the final diet, although easy to stay with, is one that you *must* stay with for a long while. No miracles are going to occur that will allow you to eat anything, or drink all sorts of caffeine, one month after you have begun this program. It won't be difficult to stay on the program, however, because you're going to feel so much better.

Trying to control the emotional situations in your life when you don't feel physically fit is extremely difficult, and fraught with hazard. Until you're thinking clearly, and this may mean three or four weeks of dieting, you shouldn't even contemplate any radical changes in your life. You may well find that as your strength returns your ability to deal with your present situations is such that there is no need to change any of them. However, if the situations are basically unmanageable, and after carefully and objectively looking at them there is nothing you can do to improve them, you'd better remove them. This might mean a new job —but are you prepared for one? Very few of us have endowments or large inheritances, and we had better

be prepared for any job change we are thinking of mak
ing. A job of lessened responsibility often looks appeal
ing, superficially. It's very dangerous to try to step too
far down from one's present levels of responsibility, far
better to gear the body machine up so it can meet
higher levels. Stepping too far down can be like racing
an engine without a load; it will explode. That same
engine could run just as fast carrying a load and be in
no danger.

Marital problems frequently spring from fatigue
and can be solved readily once the fatigue is controlled.
In this day of the young, beautiful people, you are apt
to look unappealing to your partner if you're greatly
overweight and tired all the time. This can lead to a
great deal of disharmony, which is readily corrected
when your pep and shape return.

Exercise is just as important to any diet routine as
is food. A minimum program of exercise, such as the
one outlined, will speed up your return to normal
greatly. Also, it will give you the full level of mental
and physical functioning that you are entitled to.

> *What I do for my good today*
> *will give me a better tomorrow*
> *and the best of life.*

20

Sex Failures

ONE OF the primary causes of an inability to achieve orgasm—male or female—is hypoglycemia, and its opposite number diabetes. For those with unrecognized disease these failures can be a disguised blessing, because they can cause a visit to the physician, resulting in treatment of the metabolic problem, which will increase both sexual ability and longevity.

Too often, people attempt to relate these failures to their age, believing that they are "worn-out" sexually. This old falsehood is so deeply ingrained in our entire civilization that it is probably the most effective "Big Lie" around today. Medical research continues to emphasize that sexual activity to the tenth decade of life is the norm for healthy individuals—but the lie keeps on.

Sex is as much psychologic as physical. Most of us know too little about either aspect of our sexual abilities or inabilities. The primary inability that a man complains about is difficulty in obtaining a satisfactory erection—impotence. This prevents orgasm totally. Women complain of a lack of orgasm as a primary difficulty, but the physical basis for the problem is the same as the male's. This may sound terribly surprising, unless you know the physical similarities between the male and female sexual anatomy. The names are different, the appearance—at maturity is different —but the origins of these anatomic parts are the same, just as are the difficulties. The precise way in which hypoglycemia, and other disorders, cause this is not fully understood, but correcting the bodily disease will correct the difficulty.

Both the male and female reproductive systems start originally, in the embryo, from germinal ridges at the fourth to sixth week of development. At that time a structure, the genital eminence appears. A urethral fold appears and develops differently, depending on the chromosomes of the embryo; if male, this forms the shaft of the penis; if female the labia minus—the small lips next to the vagina. Since the dawn of time mankind has been aware that this area, in the male, would—under stimulation—retain blood and cause an erection of the penis. Only recently, with the work of Masters and Johnson, has the similarity of function been shown in the female's labia minus—they also enlarge and elongate under stimulation.

When the internal machinery that regulates this blood flow to the area doesn't work, the ability for orgasm is lost. Nervousness, apprehension, as well as hypoglycemia, will sometimes cause an inability of these organs to obtain their necessary erection. In other instances, there will be a partial filling because of an inability to respond to stimulation, or because of inadequate stimulation. In the male this still prevents intercourse, in both it prevents orgasm. Even when the stimulation is quite adequate there may be a sudden loss of size because of mental or physical factors. This always seems catastrophic, and usually leads to a self-fulfilling feeling that orgasm will never be obtainable, but, fortunately, that prophecy can be changed.

Sexual over-activity, although less common, usually stems from the same causes, because it, too, represents a search for a satisfying orgasm that is not achieved. In these cases, though, the person feels that it is not their sexual difficulty, but that of their partner that is causing the trouble, and doesn't realize that their physical health—often hypoglycemia—is the root of their problem. This leads to madly promiscuous behavior with all sorts of complications and entanglements that cause more grief and more disorder as time goes on. As I have sat with various patients and discussed this problem, I at first felt the trouble was largely psychological, not a matter of any dietary error. But, as I took a complete history, I noticed there was great irregularity in eating and a strong emphasis on carbohydrate and alcohol—a speedy way to get hypoglycemia! Since these men and women were often rushing about trying to maintain "appearances" in one quarter and comradery in another, this seemed much more to be a cause than an effect.

Joan R. told me her story which was basically the same as that of her "sisters" in this problem. She was 32, attractive, bright, and very unhappy. She was married to a man she thought she still loved—but she was sexually desperate. She could achieve orgasms herself, but never in intercourse with her husband. She admitted that some of this might be her fault, but felt the majority of the trouble was with him. We talked matters over, I instructed her in playing a more active role, she had been extremely passive, and suggested some variety in their sexual approaches. This was all duly tried, failed, and reported back to me. Along with this report came a manifesto from Joan saying that she was going to go out and find herself another man, since the fault must be entirely her husband's. What she was really telling me, I felt, was I'd better hurry up and find out what was really wrong.

Joan was a flirt, and as an attractive young woman working in an office filled with men she did have many friends. No, she really didn't have her eye on anyone in particular, she just knew that when she made up her mind to switch from flirting to reality she wouldn't have much trouble in choosing her lover. We talked on and discussed her energy—nervous, yes—but pepless. I began to wonder if perhaps one physical disorder that I hadn't yet turned up was causing both this fatigue and her frustration. I prescribed further tests; the initial ones had all seemed all right. We checked the endocrine glands, because when one is off all the others tend to get somewhat out of kilter, too. Her thyroid was fine, her adrenals fine; but, her three-hour blood sugar curve looked a little peculiar. We then sat down and talked things over again getting a fuller and much more revealing story about her dietary habits. Joan really didn't know what a balanced meal was and she didn't like cooking very much, either. I gave her some instruction on diet, told her I wanted her to have the five-hour blood sugar test the next week, and sent her away in a more relaxed frame of mind. She had that test, we straightened out her hypoglycemia, and everything else clicked into place.

Men frequently ask me if they have a menopause the same way women do. No they don't, is always my answer. What they are telling me is that they are having the "Crisis of the Middle-Aged male." This is an all-too-common picture of behavior stemming from a mild desperation. Often this has been caused by their wife's menopause, and her saying, "we're too old for sex." Her attitude, of course, is based on misinformation. Many women find more pleasure, sometimes even their first pleasure, in sex after menopause. The threat of child bearing is often a hindrance, consciously or subconsciously, to full sexual pleasure. Once this threat is removed the majority of women are happier and freer in their sexuality. Many couples should be asked again to realize that sex is not everything in marriage—it comes in third! The most important factor in any marriage is companionship; friendly and loving compassion. Communication is the number two need of a happy and successful relationship. Companionship and communication usually start out high in a marriage, but too frequently disappear as habits get fixed, work increases and social obligations mount. Sex has often become, by middle-age, a routine with rigid boundaries of activity and action.

Striving for success in every way is often reflected in the thought that each and every encounter should culminate in coitus—and mutual orgasm. In a proper loving, but playful relationship this will occur, but in a striving, over-achieving pursuit toward this goal it often doesn't—can't—happen. The combination of hypoglycemia and a "calendar psychosis" often result in a sex crisis. The Kinsey Report says that there is a decline in sexual activity in most men in their forties and fifties. Most men shrug it off realizing they cannot be the same athletes they were in their twenties and thirties. Some, however, show all kinds of symptoms—the so-called male-climacterium: insecurity, general inadequateness, shame, envious of young men and often frantic attempts to assert themselves. This is when the decline becomes a fall, and the man who is not really old "gives up" on sex. Usually, with hypoglycemia and obesity, he is in poor condition for anything, including sex. There is also his state of mind. His sexual energy is being pushed aside by the worries of his disease— and he takes these worries to bed with him.

Enforced sexual abstinence is often the result of the wife's menopause and the husband's own problems.

Yes, hypoglycemia can belong to both partners in a marriage, and often does. The dietary indiscretions of the wife are almost always fed to the husband, and he may even do worse when he's on his own at lunch. This combination causes many middle-aged catastrophies. Enforced sexual abstinence in men is associated with a marked decline in the production of their hormones, according to a recent study reported at Vanderbilt University. When a man stops giving his sex glands the message to get ready for action, they apparently lose the habit. Bergler, in the Revolt of the Middle-Aged Man, says that some middle-aged men pass through a transitory period of second emotional adolescence. It may occur in the mid- or late-forties, and again in the mid-sixties. We can see, however, that mere birthdays do not change sexual interest, nor do they vanquish sexual effectiveness.

To quote Masters and Johnson, they state that the orgasm of both male and female continue well into the eighth, ninth and tenth decades of life. Infidelity often occurs at this time in an effort to solve sexual problems. Actualities of human behavior must be given weight, the rightness or wrongness of such behavior should be considered secondarily. Kinsey reported that 26 percent of women and 50 percent of the men whom he studied had experienced extramarital coitus by age 40. This does not solve sexual problems, although it occasionally provides temporary reduction in tension. Sexual success for an impotent male, or an unable female, builds up feelings of worth, but it increases resentment for the spouse. Hostile relationships at home are increased as a result of these experiences.

Other couples who are obviously both happy and loving together will agree to permit sexual experience outside of marriage—as they would a dinner or a concert with a friend. Within this definition of the marriage contract such behavior could not be called infidelity.

Straightening out your hypoglycemia may not end your sexual problems, but there is a treatment recommended by Dr. J. Dudley Chapman of Ohio which I have found to be effective both for impotence and inability. He treated a group of 74 couples by having them abstain from intercourse for three to eight weeks. Each couple was instructed to pet, fondle, and to be aroused in other ways, but in no circumstances to have intercourse. In addition, the husband could not let his wife be aware of an erection, or anything else that would make her feel any demand. During the abstinence period the woman and her husband were seen in weekly interviews, were counseled about sex, and encouraged to talk to each other about their physical and emotional requirements. After mutual respect and understanding of sexual responses developed, and the couples had an awakened desire, they were allowed to engage in intercourse. Of the patients studied, 4 out of 5 had an improved sexual life and were able to have erections and orgasms. Most of the failures occurred when the husbands refused to abstain. The best results occurred when husband and wife were able to discuss their problems and cooperate.

Both men and women can do a great deal toward heightening their sexual abilities and pleasures by *training* for orgasm. These muscular exercises, which were taught to Masters and Johnson by prostitutes, are still the most satisfactory method, according to their re-search work. These involve tensing the muscles that surround the rectum, the vagina and the bottom of the bladder—levator ani and pubo-coccygeus. We normally hold these muscles under slight tension, and deliber-ately relax them in the process of emptying our bladder and bowel. You don't have to have any special training in Yoga muscle control in order to be able to contract these muscles more vigorously than normally. At first this should be done only momentarily for a minute or two, two or three times a day. If you try to do more than that early in your muscle training program, you're apt to get a most uncomfortable cramp. Don't worry about losing control of your bowel or bladder, you will not over-relax the muscles as long as you don't over-exercise them at first. After a few such sessions you can use these muscles actively and voluntarily during the course of coitus, enhancing the pleasure for your part-ner and yourself.

One old, but still regularly published, marriage man-ual advises couples with sexual difficulties to distract themselves by thinking of something unrelated to sexual activity during coitus. This was false when it was pub-lished, but now it is so well publicized, and frequently believed, it should show us all how effective the Big Lie technique is. Distraction, or inattention, lessens the pleasure and effectiveness of loving. Undue focus on one particular part of the body can be over-exciting, but thinking of milk bills or electronic diagrams is fool-ish and beneath any couple truly in love.

There are those who have fallen "out of love," but remain married. Many marriages are outgrown. One physician recently observed that 25 years of marriage should be grounds for divorce, pointing out that this was a full life expectancy during the millennia when marriage was a promise for a "life time." Divorce is certainly not a unique idea; one out of four American marriages end in this fashion. I do not recommend it as an easy or only solution, but its existence is a fact, which some people are fearful of admitting, even to themselves. Love is the safest investment in the world, nearly everyone gets out tenfold what they put in.

21

The New
Mind Power

THE HUMAN brain is a goal-directed machine. This means that the coming events of our lives do cast their shadows before them, but we cause these shadows with our thoughts. Psychology, psychiatry and neuroanatomy have joined forces in what some call the new Copernican revolution—Thought Control. But the thought control is not done by Big Brother, it's done by

you in the way you look at yourself today and for tomorrow. You know the truth of the old cliché, Success
Breeds Success and Failure Causes Failure, through
your own experience. When you are succeeding—in
business, love, whatever—your success gives you a ra-
diant glow that attracts more success, even success of
the same order. And when "luck" is turned against you
there are those days you can't seem to do anything
right.

The times you can do nothing wrong, or nothing
right, are really self-determined times because your
luck, your happiness or whatever you want to call it,
depends more on the aim that you give your brain and
your mood than it does on anything else in the whole
world. I'm not saying that this is a new and magic way
to run your machine without gasoline, it's not. Your
own body machine can't run right when you're hypoglycemic. You have the blues, you feel so bad you do
tell yourself you can't succeed, and you're right! Hypoglycemia is giving you a habit, a habit of failure, and
just correcting the hypoglycemia won't instantly correct all your bad habits. You have to know how to
correct your habits just as much as you have to know
how to correct your diet. Now you can also know that
correcting your habits will give you just as much mental
health as correcting your diet gives you physical health.
The mental habits of hypoglycemia are what we usually
call "the blues," or if they are bad enough depression.

Depression can be a very serious disease resulting in
suicide. When I was in medical school I was taught that
people who talked about or threatened suicide never
meant it; they were just trying to get attention. Today,

all physicians know that such people *do* mean it, they are seeking attention, they are crying for help. "Stop me from doing this to myself!" A person this deep in depression needs immediate medical care, and, if possible, psychiatric help.

The blues, depression, are as different from one person to another as your fingerprint is different from mine. To one person it may be a sudden feeling of unreality—"as if everything were floating." To another it might be a feeling of estrangement and detachment from your immediate environment—"as if I were on the outside looking in." Feelings of hopelessness and helplessness are apt to be frequent. Successful men and women, the over-achievers, often feel that their success is meaningless when a depression interrupts their life. Slowing and hesitancy of thought is not unusual, and crying jags certainly occur.

Homosexual behavior, one of today's growing suburban problems, may be part of a depression, or it may cause it. Feelings of fear and unworthiness are often part of this picture and make matters worse. Futility and a feeling of the repetitiousness of life can grow into a serious depression when left to run unchecked.

You can live in a world of creative fulfillment instead of a world of destruction and depression.

How can you do it?

First, you should create and sustain higher expectations about your life. We should feel that as we grow from childhood to adulthood we are moving further toward becoming fully mature, wise, compassionate and loving individuals. We need to know that old age is not coming our way at fifty or at sixty—old age today is somewhere way past eighty. And that old age does not include senile breakdowns. With proper planning, you can create for yourself a new and far more enticing image of adulthood.

The human mind at forty commonly is vulgar, smug, deadened and wastes its hours. William Sheldon has called this the "dying back of the brain." "The days of youth teem with fragments of living knowledge; with daring philosophies; morning dreams; plans. . . . Everywhere adult brains seem to resemble blighted trees that have died in the upper branches, yet cling to the struggling green wisps of life about the lower trunk." (William H. Sheldon, *Psychology and the Promethean Will,* Harper and Row, N.Y.)

This is a too-common, and awfully uninspiring image of adult years. It's the image that many of the young have, and probably the reason they say, "trust no one over thirty." Your extended middle years should have an increasing power and sense of fulfillment, rather than a dampening down, a letting go or making the best of things.

What is adulthood? Harry Stack Sullivan, M.D. wrote: "I believe that for a great majority of our people preadolescence is the nearest they come to untroubled human life—from then on the stresses of life distort them into inferior caricatures of what they might have been." The processes and powers that we have trained in youth, and developed during our early years, should come to fruition as we acquire age and wisdom unless our eyes are closed to everything. The good news that life grows in powers and happiness by linking itself productively to other lives, increasing knowledge, increasing responsibility, through empathy, through sexual understanding, and through philosophy is the message of the joy of our life. With this there is no necessary road to adult dullness, no fatal "dying back of the brain." The blues happen too often because of the feeling of waste and disappointment in our adult years. The reason is found in those conditions which have halted your growing with life and are breaking your linkage with life. These conditions don't have to exist; if they do you can alter them. You can create conditions far more favorable than ever before for the growth of your life into a maturity that is a triumph.

Life is filled with choices, and as we make them moment by moment, we direct ourselves toward joy or despair. You do not have to wait for a special moment to make a decision about your moods and your enjoyment of life—those moments are occurring continually.

For example, in business or at home someone will make a mistake. This can be an occasion for an angry scolding, merciless mocking, or an abrupt dismissal of that person. Or it can be an occasion for recognizing the human capacity we all have to make mistakes, and working around them.

The adult male fascination for baseball and football, I think, stems from this desire to know and see the mistakes of others. They feel reassured when the best hitter in the league averages out to making little more than one hit for every three times at bat. Such a ball player is idolized and lionized, but with a certain secret satisfaction that he's not Superman—just a very good ball player.

To some, marriage means a continual active combative experience with their spouse. At the other end of the scale it means so much mutuality of interests and actions that neither person feels complete without the other. Unfortunately battles or indifferent tolerance seem to be more the rule of marriages than total harmony. Kinsey reported, and other researchers have recently agreed, that about 40 percent of married women *do not* love their husbands! A relationship like this is apt to be terribly damaging for both parties, and it certainly can lead to a logical and total depression. The maintenance of marriage for social reasons is certain to spell disaster, at least for one party, and often for both. Children should not be raised in such an environment, any more than they should be physically beaten. The scars and injuries that warring parents inflict upon their children's developing psyche through lovelessness and selfishness can often only be corrected in latter years through extensive psychiatric counselling, if then.

The war between the generations is not at all new to our time. Socrates pointed it out, as did Babylonian writers 1500 years before him. In particular households this usually begins when the adolescent member of the family starts bringing home opinions other than those that have been standard for the family. This can lead to frequent occasions where the adults express their shock and disapproval, point out the ridiculousness of the danger of these views, and warn the adolescent that he needs to grow up, as his parents have. Or it can lead to occasions when the adults sit down and talk it out with the adolescent getting a full expression of his views, "listening with real interest, expressing honest doubts about his position and their own, but expressing them in such a way that the youth is given to feel that he has a right to a mind of his own." Answering all their arguments may seem difficult, or even impossible, but usually the youth does not so much want his arguments answered as listened to so that he can "chew them over" himself, knowing that he has made a step toward mature communication with his parents in the process. Today, when the size of the younger generation is so huge that it has become its own sub-culture, the feeling of aloneness is even greater for them. Depression and suicide is prevalent in this group, particularly among the high achievers. Yet, many of these depressions would have no ground to grow upon had there been communication, not necessarily agreement, between parents and youth.

In Boston there is a tablet in front of the Old South Meeting House which says our Revolutionary forefathers were "worthy to raise issues." The necessity of mature and thoughtful judgment before raising issues still persists, although too many individuals in their middle years feel that they can only trust those over forty. Too often, what they mean is they don't wish to raise any issues, because that will incur some danger, even when the voice of protest needs to be raised. Last year in Detroit at a series of interracial meetings, one of the chief executives of the Ford Company was continually delighted by the thoughtful and very profound comments of one of the black leaders. And he was greatly amazed when he found out, after several lengthy meetings, that this individual was eighteen years old!

Extreme youth and extreme age are no barrier to intelligent and mature thought. Too many of us forget that Alexander the Great had reached the ripe old age of twenty-three when he complained he had no more worlds to conquer. Disraeli was an ordinary tailor until he was past sixty-five; then his time arrived to be a leader of an empire greater than Alexander's.

Who are your friends and acquaintances? They are the ones who will give you the blues or joy. We all know that there are groups that perpetuate various immaturities, groups whose only significance is their snobbishness or exclusiveness, those that turn life into perpetual self-indulgence, groups that preach love, but practice intolerance, groups that require undeviating partisan loyalty. Or are your friends in those groups that significantly work toward maturity, groups that deliberately seek to overcome prejudices, racial, social and other, even though that work is often dangerous; groups that encourage citizenship by active work for community betterment and awareness of the critical issues. If you're one who "gives a damn" about poverty, ignorance, slum life, unemployment, discrimination, the very meaningfulness of your involvement will give you a richer life and one far from the blues.

Real, active involvement with a voluntary group is today's area where the individual can enlarge his own lesser strength with the greater combined strength of those who care about fulfillment in living. In previous centuries a person of high concern would undergo the discipline of holiness. He would join a holy fellowship and under a planned discipline would work for "the glory of God." This is an older way of enlisting one's individual efforts with the efforts of a group that strove for fulfillment. This discipline of holiness has largely disappeared today, and we often go our individual ways without the sense of mission to perform and without a disciplined companionship that helps us do it. It may be that a new way of discipline is being shaped. It can be seen in the individual who, in a passion for justice for mistreated fellow mankind, spends days and nights hard at work for laws that will straighten out the injustices; or he who sees the limitations our cities place upon child life, and who works for breathing space and playing space; as well as he who seeks a better understanding of the young lives trapped in ghettoes.

This self-dedication and self-discipline takes many forms. The important thing for you is to lend yourself heart and soul to goals that go beyond your own ego-satisfaction. The time is out of joint and the call is for all good men and women to straighten it out.

One of the current fatalities bred into our culture is idolizing youth and immaturity. Youth is looked back upon wistfully as a golden time by those who view aging only as a process ending in fatality and senility—not a time of maturity. The obligations of adulthood bring with them a new significance and creative happiness that never exist in youth. The passing of youth doesn't mean slipping into a dullness of routine and to the anxieties of an economic treadmill. It should mean a new dimension in life, with zestful activity bringing new experiences rather than merely compensating for the loss of the young years.

This idolization of childhood and youth has influenced all of us. It has made parents afraid of their children, afraid to set reasonable standards for them lest the children think of them as reactionaries. It has made advertisers able to frighten us into buying almost anything that will keep us from looking old. It has also confused educational standards into a sole service of the young. Our culture does not give adults even a fraction of what schools, colleges, and universities give so generously to children and youth. All of this works against the idea of the dignity in adult living.

Adult education is still offered more often for entertainment than for transformation and accomplishment; craft work, a hobby, something to enliven or at least beguile a few hours. Stirring the mind just a very little is too often the goal of these courses. However, adulthood can be a time of growth and learning equally as fascinating as childhood. New and significant changes go on throughout our life-experience. Psychological maturing is the most triumphant way of human fulfillment, and this is only possible in the adult years. Mature insights exist which children and adolescents cannot possibly have. Reflect on your own youth—they weren't triumphant years, but years of various frustrations; more so than you have today. Can youth think mature thoughts, and do mature things? Not while they are young. George Bernard Shaw was more cynical than correct when he said that it was such a pity to waste youth on the young. Youth is the time of budding development. Full realization of life can only come in your adult years.

Although hypoglycemia got you to this state, simple correction of it alone won't get you out of all these problems. Nor can you simply *think* your way out of the problems with no attention to diet. But by feeding yourself as you should, both physically and mentally, you will become all that you ever hoped to be—because that, and only that, is the True You.

22

Your Diet Diary

BY LOOKING into your own actions, with this diary, you can pretty well determine if the Hypoglycemia diet is helping you. These little tests, and their answers written in, will give you—and your physician—a bench mark for comparisons. You should start them as you start your diet plan, either the one week, or the two week, test which ever suits you best.

DAY ONE

Just before breakast:

> Do you have a headache?
> Did you sleep well?
> Did you dream a lot?
> Do you feel dizzy or fatigued?

Before lunch:

> Have you had any episodes of weakness since breakfast?
> Are you aware of excess perspiration since breakfast?

Before mid-afternoon snack:

> How is your physical strength, now?
> Have you been shaky?
> Do you feel mentally alert?

Before dinner:

> Are you ravenously hungry now, or comfortable?
> Quickly subtract nines from 100, and see how long it takes you to get finished.

Before retiring:

> Does your tummy feel stuffed?
> Have you been going to the bathroom excessively today?
> Do the multiplication tables of 7's. How long did that take you?

DAY TWO

Before mid-morning snack:

Have you been angry at anyone this morning?

Do you feel nervous and edgy?

Do you want this snack—or does the idea upset you?

After lunch:

Did you enjoy lunch, or was something missing?

How does the afternoon line up—are you ready for it?

Say, and listen to yourself as you say "Methodist—Episcopal" three times quickly. Is your enunciation exact, or is it slurred?

After dinner:

Do you feel energetic, or do you wish to lie down?

Who is the President of Rumania?

What's 7 times 24? How long did that take?

Before retiring:

Have you had any sweating episodes today?

Do you feel like falling asleep, or are your muscles restless?

Have you noticed any changes in your vision today?

DAY THREE

Before breakfast:

> Did you sleep well last night?
> Do you feel like taking some exercizes this morning?
> Are you looking forward to today?

Before lunch:

> Have you felt happy this morning?
> Is your sense of humor returning?
> Is it easier, or harder, to make decisions now than it was a week ago?

Mid-afternoon:

> Have you had any undue perspiring today?
> Are you getting your snacks on time, or are you about one-half hour late in having them?

Mid-evening:

> What have you been doing since dinner? Are you enjoying it?
> Are you getting better at solving problems?
> 73289526—Can you remember this? Without looking at it again write it down just before you go to bed, and check it.

DAY FOUR

Just before breakfast:

Do you have a headache?
Did you sleep well?
Did you dream a lot?
Do you feel dizzy or fatigued?

Before lunch:

Have you had any episodes of weakness since breakfast?
Are you aware of excess perspiration since breakfast?

Before mid-afternoon snack:

How is your physical strength, now?
Have you been shaky?
Do you feel mentally alert?

Before dinner:

Are you ravenously hungry now, or comfortable?
Quickly subtract nines from 100, and see how long it takes you to get finished, this time.

Before retiring:

Does your tummy feel stuffed?
Have you been going to the bathroom excessively today?
Do the multiplication tables of 9's. How long did that take you?

DAY FIVE

Before mid-morning snack:

Have you been angry at anyone this
morning?

Do you feel nervous and edgy?

Do you want this snack—or does
the idea upset you?

After lunch:

Did you enjoy lunch, or was something missing?

How does the afternoon line up—
are you ready for it?

Say, and listen to yourself as you
say "Methodist—Episcopal"
three times quickly. Is your enunciation exact, or is it slurred?

After dinner:

Do you feel energetic, or do you
wish to lie down?

Who is the President of Poland?

What's 7 times 18? How long did
that take?

Before retiring:

Have you had any sweating episodes today?

Do you feel like falling asleep, or
are your muscles restless?

Have you noticed any changes in
your vision today?

DAY SIX

Before breakfast:

Did you sleep well last night?
Do you feel like taking some exercises this morning?
Are you looking forward to today?

Before lunch:

Have you felt happy this morning?
Is your sense of humor returning?
Is it easier, or harder, to make decisions now than it was a week ago?

Mid-afternoon:

Have you had any undue perspiring today?
Are you getting your snacks on time, or are you about one-half hour late in having them?
73289526—Can you remember this? Without looking at it again write it down just before you go to bed, and check it.

DAY SEVEN

Before breakfast:

How do you feel?
How did you sleep?
Did you dream—pleasant or frightening?
Have you started exercise?

Before lunch:

Has the day gone smoothly, with minor irritations, "rolling-off"?
Do you feel more alive than you did last week?

Before dinner:

Do you feel more like making plans for the future?
Do your plans include "fun" things?
Is your digestion better?
Are you better able to deal with people than you were?

GOOD HEALTH AND GOOD LUCK